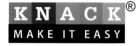

WEIGHT TRAINING
FOR WOMEN

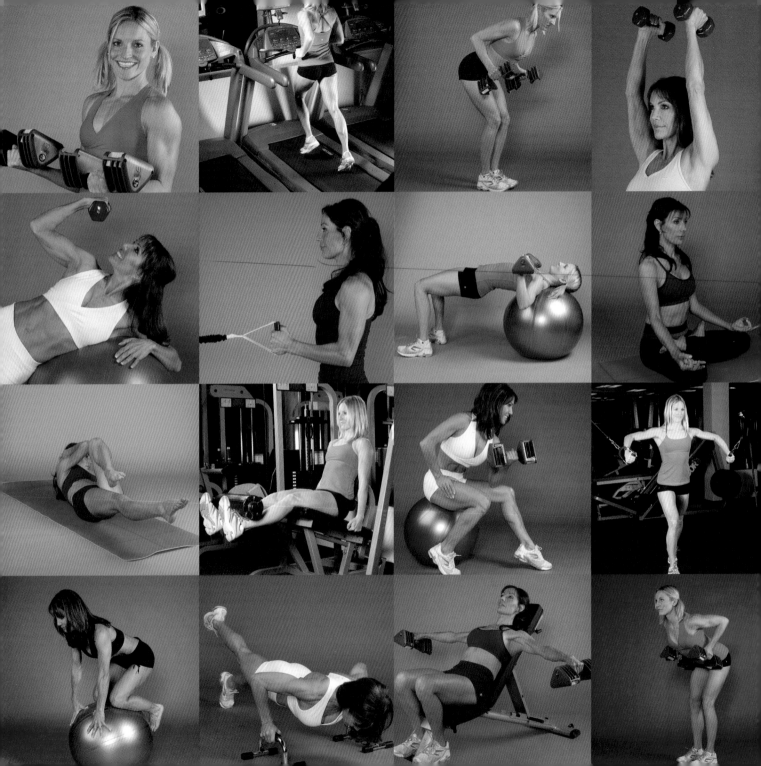

KNACK®

WEIGHT TRAINING
FOR WOMEN

Step-by-Step Exercises for Weight Loss, Body Shaping, and Good Health

LEAH GARCIA

Photographs by Mark Doolittle

Technical review by Jennifer Brindisi, B.S., M.A.

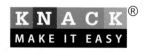

KNACK®
MAKE IT EASY

Guilford, Connecticut
An imprint of The Globe Pequot Press

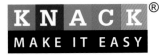

Copyright © 2009 by Morris Book Publishing, LLC

Editor in Chief: Maureen Graney
Editor: Imee Curiel
Cover Design: Paul Beatrice, Bret Kerr
Text Design: Paul Beatrice
Layout: Kevin Mak
Cover photos by Mark Doolittle
All interior photos by Mark Doolittle with the exception of p. 6
(fruits) © Barbara Helgason | Dreamstime.com and p. 12 (muscle
groups) © Bonfils Fabien | Dreamstime.com
Illustration on p. 46 by Ian Adamson © The Globe Pequot Press

Library of Congress Cataloging-in-Publication Data

Garcia, Leah.
 Knack weight training for women : step-by-step exercises for
weight loss, body shaping, and good health / Leah Garcia ; photo-
graphs by Mark Doolittle ; technical review by Jennifer Brindisi.
   p. cm.
Includes index.
ISBN 978-1-59921-562-4
 1. Women—Health and hygiene. 2. Weight training for women.
3. Physical fitness for women. 4. Weight loss. 5. Self-care, Health. I.
Title.

RA778.G338 2009
613.7'045—dc22
                              2009010786

The following manufacturers/names appearing in *Knack Weight
Training* for Women are trademarks:
Body Bars®, FreeMotion™ Fitness, Accu-Measure®, Tanita®, BOSU®,
DuraBall™, Gliding™ discs, SelectaBell™, Contour Abs™, Naturally
Caffeinated®, Yoga-Paws®

Printed in China

10 9 8 7 6 5 4 3 2 1

This book is intended as a reference guide, not as a medical
manual. The ideas, procedures, and suggestions contained herein
are not intended as a substitute for consulting with your physician.
Starting a new fitness regimen should begin with making a candid
assessment of your current health and fitness level. If you have any
questions about your health, you should consult your physician
before beginning this or any fitness program.

This book is dedicated to my mother, Patricia Urrutia-Garcia, whose eternal strength continues to lift me higher.

Acknowledgments

To all of my early mentors, coaches, fitness inspirations, and sponsors, I thank you for giving me the courage to live true to my dreams and for teaching me about dedication and being a professional. Two standout colleagues, Dale Henn and Mike Hays, have honored me with opportunities that remain unsurpassed. I am eternally grateful to be part of their lives and business ventures. I would like to extend a big thank-you to Glen Marshman, owner of One Boulder Fitness, for opening his doors to me, especially early on, as a personal trainer. For this book project, I would also like to acknowledge Jilayne Lovejoy for her guidance, and thank my models: Andrea Malmberg, esthetician; Andie Bernard, NSCA-certified personal trainer and Usana Health Sciences associate; and Sana Bridges, certified Pilates, yoga, and functional fitness instructor. Sana provided unparalleled collaboration on the exercises within this book, making it more holistic and balanced. I am overwhelmingly indebted to Ian Adamson, seven-time adventure racing world champion, the love of my life, my greatest partner, and unconditional supporter. If it weren't for him, it is doubtful that I would eat as many delicious home-cooked meals or have as much fun. Thank you all!

CONTENTS

INTRODUCTION

Have you ever noticed that the more you read about weight training and fitness, the more daunting it becomes? It seems so complicated. There are stability balls for functional fitness, heart rate monitors and their accompanying training zones, fancy gym machines, home equipment contraptions, and products that promise to drop fat and get you toned, in eight minutes a day. Health and fitness magazines need to keep the content fresh, so they feature cool exercises and new looks every month. Trying to keep up with their advice is a full-time job. Most weight training books feature so many programs and detailed information that it becomes overwhelming. Eventually what's needed is a step-by-step, no-nonsense approach that goes back to the basics, incorporating variety and holistic movement.

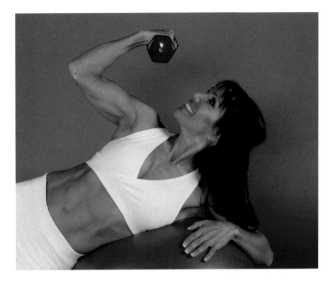

Women are happier and more confident when they lift weights

Getting physically stronger makes daily tasks easier. Healthy muscle fibers and stable joints and connective tissue equate to more protection for the body and reduced injury. A toned midsection looks good and serves a purpose. Strong abdominals, especially the deepest in the core, protect the back. In fact, back pain is often eliminated when you practice strength training. Lifting weights also increases bone mineral density, which helps fight osteoporosis. Diabetes, arthritis, and heart disease risks also are reduced from strength training. What's more, as cardiovascular condition improves, cholesterol levels become healthier. The bottom line is this: Women of all ages show improvement when they strength train. And the good news is: It's never too late to start.

If your goal is to be leaner, weight lifting is an excellent way to promote healthy fat loss. When you strength train, you build more lean body mass. The more lean muscle on your body, the more your energy and resting metabolism is increased. A higher resting metabolism means you burn more calories when you are not exercising. Your body wants to be strong. Your body was designed for action, for movement, for activity. After learning how to seamlessly incorporate weight training into your weekly routine, you will reap the benefits of your natural genetics. And no, you won't get bulky in the process.

Today you are "training"

No longer are you dieting or just going to the gym to exercise. Your code word is *training*. Personal experience has taught me that when you tell people you are training, they treat you with positive energy and respect. In the past, when I was a diet freak—and believe me, I've tried them all—it was a battle to eat with friends and family. Once the word *diet* came out of my mouth, I heard the same response over and over. "Diet? You? Why? You don't need to diet. Come on, just enjoy this dessert." The same held true when I told people exercise was my priority. "Exercise? Why? You're already fit, you can skip it today." Training intrigues people. Instead of drawing judgment,

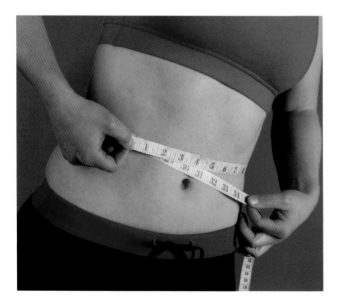

it creates conversation and reframes the focus on a goal. "What are you training for?" The answer is up to you. Some recommended responses include, "Life, career, higher energy level, a race, or an exciting occasion." I'm okay with any and all, so long as you always have a destination point in mind.

Proper lifting form is critical to success

Lifting properly allows you to stay injury free, helps your body progress, and creates a positive flow. Memorize the chapters on proper lifting form (chapter 2) and the lower abdominal muscles (chapter 5). It is important to maintain a universal body awareness and posture, which will serve you well throughout life. Generally speaking everyone needs to train the stabilizer muscles. These support your prime movers, or big muscles, and provide a foundation for posture and movement. Don't skip the detail work when training. The objective is not to lift more weight or do more push-ups. It is to make every action beautiful, flowing, biomechanically correct, and safe.

Once your core, knees, shoulders, hips, and joints are stable, more agility, flexibility, vitality, and personal gains will happen. This is the foundation for your training. You will need to distinguish between sharp, piercing pain—which is harmful—and an uncomfortable burn or mild discomfort—which at times is part of the process. At no point should you continue on with an exercise if you experience bad pain. If you have personal limitations and preexisting conditions, skip the exercises that are contraindicative.

Please check with your doctor before starting this or any personal exercise program. It would be beneficial for you to get a base-line fitness test, including a lipid profile, pulmonary lung capacity, resting heart rate, blood pressure, body composition (body mass index), girth measurement, flexibility, and cardiovascular and muscular strength and endurance test. (See chapter 1 for a more thorough explanation.) Sports medicine facilities are an excellent resource for testing.

The American College of Obstetricians and Gynecologists has given its stamp of approval to exercise during pregnancy and the postpartum period. Please work within the prenatal guidelines for your personalized program if you fall into these categories.

Hire a professional

Using a certified personal trainer or coach can be a great way to get you started in your training and ensure you adopt good habits. Start a budget for this luxury today, especially if you learn through visual, auditory, and tactile senses. This book cannot reach out and cue you when your form is suffering. A trainer or coach can help guide you, monitoring alignment and progress. Before hiring a personal trainer, be sure to research his or her accreditations. Hands-on trainers who are engaged and organized and create a customized program are recommended.

With or without gym experience, you have before you a guide with strength, heart-healthy, mind/body, agility, and wellness exercises as a reference for your daily practice at home or work and when traveling. You will find a lot of rewarding and challenging moves in this resource. The advanced images are not meant to intimidate, but to inspire you. You will find plenty of exercises to help you progress to this level. Skip the moves that you can't perform with good form, or neutral body position, and/or modify them to accommodate your fitness level. Eventually you will get there.

Make sure that early on, every workout leaves you craving the next. Push yourself enough to feel energized and vital, not thrashed. More advanced training will challenge the body with greater specificity and intensity. Chapter 18 has a body-shaping split routine that is very difficult. Save this workout for a time when you have eight weeks to focus and you feel confident that your body is capable of handling the workload.

This is not a nutrition book

There are two pages in this book that cover nutrition, diet, fat loss, and cellulite. Honor the experts and your doctor when it comes to your nutritional requirements. Use common sense and listen to the kind voice in your head prompting you to drink plenty of water, eat as much organic, healthy fruits and vegetables as possible,

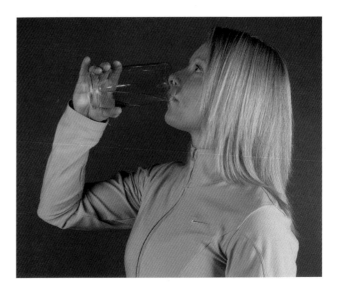

and consume sufficient protein. If you eat packaged and processed foods, trans fats may be lurking (not good for your health!). For those on a diet, the golden rule applies: Calories in—calories out. Burn more calories than you consume, and you will drop weight.

Be Naturally Caffeinated

To be Naturally Caffeinated is a state of high energy, enthusiasm, and enjoyment of life. It is a term used to describe individuals who energize their bodies and their lives through movement, activity, and healthy living. I have distilled my lifetime of knowledge on strength training, fitness, and practical sense into this book so that you can create your own personal practice and develop healthy habits—which will last a lifetime.

Being fit and healthy will make it possible to seize the moment, whenever that moment presents itself. Are you ready? It's time to "wake up your potential"!

Leah Garcia
Founder
Naturally Caffeinated, Inc.

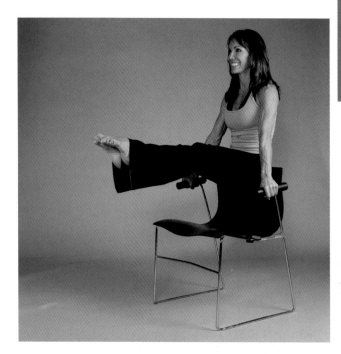

WHY LIFT WEIGHTS?

You will increase strength, lose body fat, reduce health risks, and improve your attitude

Lifting weights will not make you bulk up. Women do not have enough of the hormone testosterone to get big muscles. Because muscle takes up less space than fat in the body, women tend to *lose* inches when they strength train. By adding more lean muscle, they tone up instead of bulk up.

There are other compelling reasons to lift weights. You will become physically stronger, and daily activities will become easier. If carrying your children, moving household items, or getting up and down causes you to fatigue, more muscular strength and fitness is your solution.

Research has found that weight training can help your body ward off disease. For one, it contributes to increased

Weight Lifting

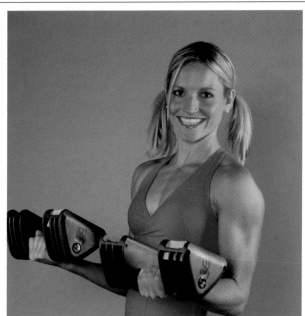

- Women excel when they have purpose; a personal mission beyond family and work keeps women emotionally, mentally, and physically lifted.

- Femininity is not compromised by having a strong, muscular physique.

- Every added pound of lean muscle, achieved through weight training, burns an additional 30 to 50 calories each day.

Resistance Bar Training

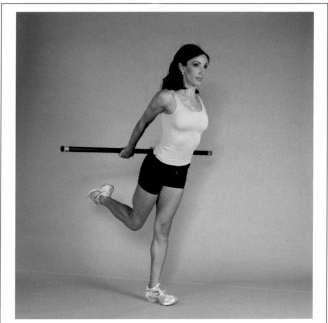

- Women respond to balance exercises, primarily because they are good at it!

- Positive reinforcement is a key element to success for training programs.

- The better you get at an activity, the more enthusiastic you are to repeat it.

- It is never too late to start lifting weights.

bone mineral density, helping to fight osteoporosis. Diabetes, arthritis, and heart disease risks are reduced with strength training, too. Your body will become more efficient—it will process sugar better and develop stronger connective tissue. Your cardiovascular health will also improve, as regular exercise helps lower bad LDL cholesterol and increases the good HDL kind. Weight lifting also decreases back pain and the risk of injury as your body develops more stability.

ZOOM

Studies performed by Wayne Westcott, Ph.D., from the South Shore YMCA in Quincy, Massachusetts, found that the average woman who strength trains two to three times a week for two months will gain nearly 2 pounds of muscle and will lose 3.5 pounds of fat.

Feeling Good

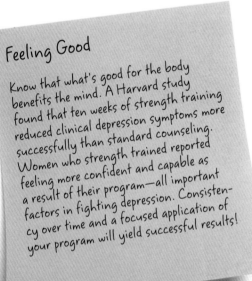

Know that what's good for the body benefits the mind. A Harvard study found that ten weeks of strength training reduced clinical depression symptoms more successfully than standard counseling. Women who strength trained reported feeling more confident and capable as a result of their program—all important factors in fighting depression. Consistency over time and a focused application of your program will yield successful results!

Life Training

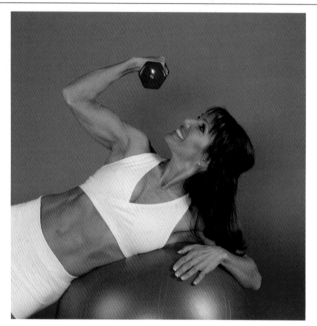

- Lifting weights should be fun. There is no reason not to smile, laugh, joke, and have a good time while training.

- You can train at home or in a fitness center or gym.

- Enjoy each moment of working your muscles the way they are intended to be used.

CARDIO AND CROSS-TRAINING

Strengthen your heart, burn calories, increase endurance, and stay motivated with more variety

Cardiovascular training, also called aerobic exercise, has to do with the heart and respiratory system. The respiratory system takes in oxygen; oxygen enters the bloodstream through your lungs; and the red blood cells in the body carry oxygen from your lungs to the tissues.

Cardio training burns fat and helps keep it off your body. Non-weight-bearing exercises are low impact and include swimming, cycling, and machines like ellipticals and recumbent and stationary bikes. These are great choices for people who are overweight, lack conditioning, or have joint issues. Weight-bearing exercise—working your body weight against gravity—is high impact and includes running and stair climbing.

Treadmill

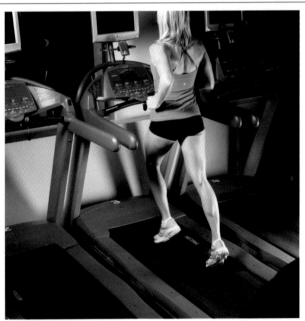

- Walking and running will strengthen your skeletal support muscles and your heart and help maintain bone mass, which prevents osteoporosis.

- Treadmills provide time-efficient training, delivering results in less time and effort.

- Keep your heart rate elevated and work up a sweat during each workout.

Elliptical Trainer

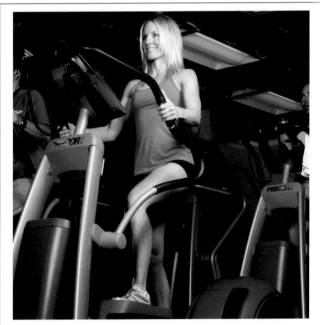

- Elliptical machines combine a natural, fluid motion of walking or cross-country skiing.

- This low-impact form of cardio exercise is easy on knees, hips, and back and will strengthen and tone legs and arms.

- Twenty minutes per session is effective to improve heart health and burn calories.

Cross-training refers to a combination of two or more types of physical activity. This is an alternative to training via a repetitive activity. Cross-training helps keep you interested in exercise, giving your mind, muscles, and joints a break from repetitive stresses.

Aim for training the cardiovascular system a minimum of three—and up to six—days a week, ideally for twenty to sixty minutes per session. The shorter the duration, the more intensity you should incorporate. If you can't carry on a conversation, but can maintain the pace, you'll burn maximum calories.

········· GREEN ● LIGHT ·········

To get more from a treadmill workout, use the quick-start setting and vary the speed manually for interval training. Warm up for ten minutes at 4 miles per hour (mph). Increase speed to 5.5 or 6.0 mph and jog for five minutes. Continue increasing speed by 0.5 mph until you reach your goal, for example 7.5 to 8.0 mph, then decrease speed by 0.5 mph until you return to your starting speed. Flat track (no incline) is recommended for this routine.

Heart Rate Monitor

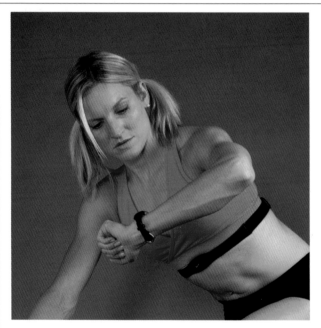

- Heart rate monitors are ideal for assessing cardiovascular condition and gauging the level of intensity of exercise.

- Heart rate monitors come in many shapes and sizes. The chest strap, which fits under breasts and bra, is very accurate and transmits the heart rate to a wristwatch.

Indoor Cycling

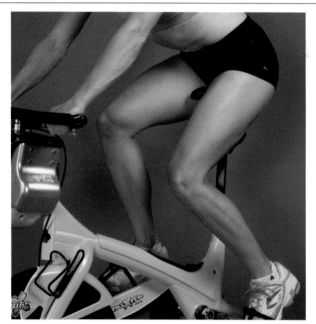

- Indoor cycling as a form of cardio training works quadriceps, hamstrings, hips, calves, and abs.

- Indoor cycling classes are offered at most clubs. A forty-minute workout, three times a week will rapidly improve your fitness.

- With group activities, don't push beyond your comfort zone just to keep up with the class.

CELLULITE AND "SPOT REDUCING"

Diet, exercise, and massage are your best weapons against cellulite; not creams, gels, or drugs

Cellulite is a condition that affects about 90 percent of American women to some degree. While it is most visible in the obese population, thin women can also display cellulite. It is a condition caused by the composition and behavior of your fat cells and the connective tissue that holds them in place. As you gain weight, the fat cells expand and bulge toward the surface of the skin, creating a bumpy appearance. This is partly due to the fact that woman have very inflexible connective tissue and *thin skin*.

Estrogen and other hormones play a dominant role in the formation of cellulite. Genetic factors, including gender, race, hormone receptors, and circulatory insufficiency, are causes

Diet and Exercise

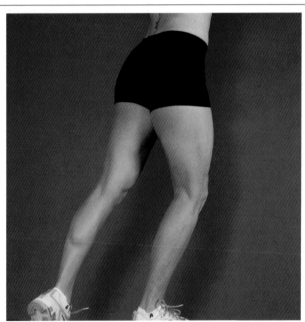

- Spot reducing is a myth.

- To lose body fat, you must train all the muscles of your body with weights, engage in cardiovascular exercise, and follow a clean diet of high-fiber foods, lean protein sources, fruits and vegetables, and plenty of water.

Hips and Thighs

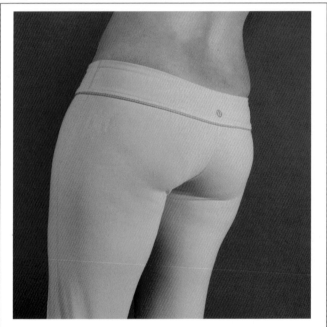

- A healthy body-fat range for a female between the ages of thirty and thirty-nine years old is between18 and 22 percent.

- Creams, gels, supplements, and pharmacological agents have not been shown to effectively work on cellulite.

- Mesotherapy, liposuction, and expensive medical procedures are not reliable methods for treating the problem.

that you cannot control. However, you can minimize cellulite with good habits. Smoking, stress, and long periods of sitting all contribute to the creation of cellulite. Diet, exercise, and massage are your best weapons to combat the problem. Avoid excess dietary fat, especially trans fats, and empty, nutritionally poor carbohydrates like cookies and chips. Reduce your salt intake and make sure to eat plenty of high-fiber, healthy foods. Weight and cardio training will reduce your total body fat, helping to tone and smooth out the skin.

· · · · · · · · · · · RED ● LIGHT · · · · · · · · · · ·

Without exercise you will lose an average of 5 pounds of muscle per decade before menopause and 1 pound a year thereafter. This muscle loss leads to a metabolic rate reduction of 2 to 5 percent per decade, and calories that were once used for muscle energy are put into fat storage and cellulite caches. Muscle mass also supports skin; when it deteriorates, you're left with a saggy, lumpy void.

Electromuscle Stimulation

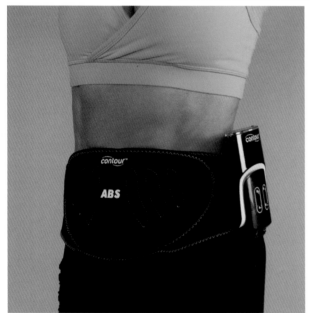

- Contour Abs electromuscle stimulation (e-stim), a Class II medical device cleared by the FDA, is a form of strength-training exercise.

- E-stim will tone and strengthen without psycho-logical or muscular fatigue, allowing for longer, perfect workouts.

- More lean muscle mass helps weight and fat loss.

Weighted Side Crunches

Don't do this!

- Avoid side bending with weights. Doing so creates thicker abs.

- Rotating movements slim the waist.

- To lose 1 pound of body weight, create a 3,500-calorie deficit through a combination of diet and exercise.

- Calorie calculators are available to determine calories burned.

NUTRITION

Drink water when you feel tired and hungry, as our signals are often confused

Steps must be taken in your current life to provide long-term benefits to your health and heart. Don't eat more calories than you can burn in a day, eat a variety of nutritious foods from all food groups, and drink plenty of water. Eat small meals, preferably four to six per day, to maintain elevated energy, metabolism, and mood and to keep your blood sugar in balance.

A realistic method to maintain balance involves a three-to-one ratio of good eating to sloppy habits. This means that if you eat well 75 percent of the time, you have a 25 percent "slop" factor for special occasions. It is not scientific, but this method does provide an attainable goal.

We eat for many reasons that do not involve hunger. For

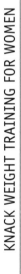
Healthy Nutrition

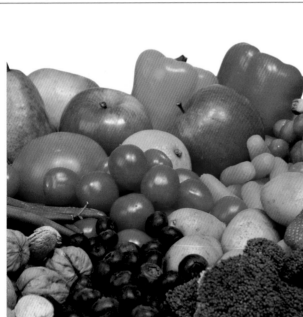

- Consuming a variety of natural or organic, nutrient-rich fruits, vegetables, and nuts is recommended for nutritional value.

- Avoid simple and processed carbohydrates (packaged sweets) and produce that has been treated with pesticides and insecticides.

- All dietary surpluses are converted to fat. Don't overeat!

Nutrition Label

- The serving size determines the calories and nutrients shown on a label.

- Serving size may be smaller than you expect.

- Avoid products with partially hydrogenated oils, as these trans fats are toxic (poison to the body) and will make you fat.

example, being tired may cause you to eat sugary foods and carbohydrates as a means to generate energy. This creates emotional ups and downs; plus it adds extra calories to the day's allotment. Always drink water when you think you're hungry, waiting a bit before eating. When you do eat, try to include a lean protein source and healthy fat to keep your body satiated.

Take a supplement if you are not able to consume enough essential fatty acids and amino acids in your diet. Always choose organic and natural over processed foods.

YELLOW LIGHT

The right number of calories to eat each day is based on your age, physical activity level, and whether you are trying to gain, lose, or maintain weight. You have the freedom to derive your daily allotment of calories based on high-calorie, nutritionally poor foods and beverages if you want. Just understand the consequences of these actions if this is the route you choose.

Water

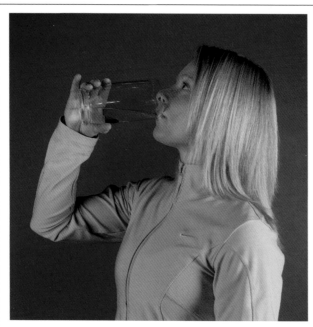

- Up to 70 percent of our body is water.

- How much water you need depends on many factors, including your health status, activity, and environ-

ment. Aim for eight to ten glasses a day.

- Drink before you are thirsty. Dehydration makes you grumpy and sleepy and causes headaches.

Protein

Dietary protein is necessary to build and repair tissue and to carry out metabolic processes. The body may use protein as an energy source when the preferred carbohydrate and fat supplies run low. The average adult woman requires 1 gram of protein per 2.2 pounds of body weight per day, or the equivalent of 70 grams per day. Depending on your activity level, this number may be higher.

ENERGY, RECOVERY, SLEEP

Who couldn't use improved focus, better flexibility, more energy, and happiness every day?

Exercise and weight training will give you energy, boost your immune system, and help your state of mind. Endorphins, released during and after exercise, are opiate-like hormones manufactured by the body. They contribute to feelings of well-being.

If you are sedentary or unfit, build up your fitness so that

with each session you feel more capable, in control, and proud of your accomplishments. Initially you may feel less than euphoric during exercise, but eventually you will get there. Too much, too soon may cause burnout.

If you are fit you are at risk of overtraining. This occurs when you consistently train too much or too often, or when you

Towel Stretch

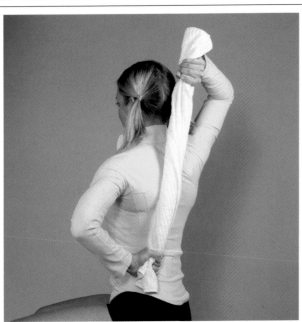

- Stretching helps with recovery by facilitating blood and nutrient flow to the muscles and helping to eliminate waste products.

- Muscle fibers and connective tissue that are stifled

and have lost their pliability inhibit repair. This is not good.

- Stretching increases muscle length and improves flexibility.

Energy and Vitality

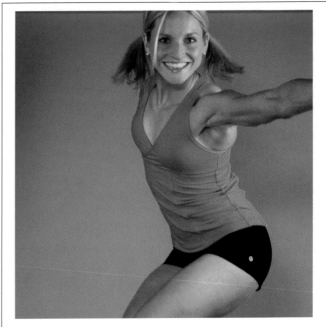

- Avoid habits that sabotage your goals. Repeatedly saying, "I'm tired," or "I don't feel well," will manifest that experience.

- Try saying, "I will feel better soon," when not at your optimum.

- Eat well, sleep sufficiently, and train with balance. Your body, mood, and intellect will reward you.

fail to get enough recovery in between workouts. Overtraining can cause chronic fatigue, insomnia, injury, illness, and changes in appetite.

You may have to explore what works for you when balancing energy, recovery, and exercise. Keeping a journal is helpful to monitor daily and weekly changes, as it provides instant feedback. A journal also creates accountability and aids motivation.

To help with post-workout recovery, eat a protein-rich meal or snack with complex carbohydrates. Protein shakes with fruit are a great option.

Massage

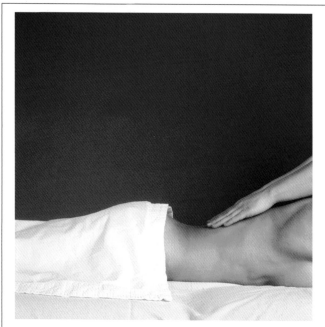

- Massage reduces stress, depression, and anxiety.

- Massage diminishes body pain, improves range of motion, enhances the immune system, stretches muscles, improves the condition of the skin, and helps with joint flexibility.

- It pumps oxygen into tissues and vital organs, helping circulation and reducing scar tissue adhesions.

Sleep

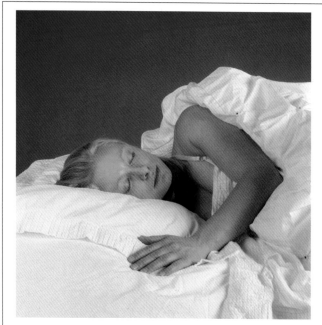

- After a workout, allow at least three or four hours before bedtime.

- The bedroom should only be used for sleep and intimacy, not watching television, eating, or reading.

- Eating a large meal or drinking caffeinated beverages before bedtime can cause sleep disorders.

- A 10- to 20-minute midday power nap rejuvenates body and mind.

FITNESS ASSESSMENT, GOAL SETTING

If you don't know where you're going, how are you going to get there?

Starting with a comprehensive fitness assessment allows you to obtain information needed to safely and effectively develop an individualized exercise program. This baseline information allows pre-test and post-test comparisons and an accurate gauge of your progress. A good gym will have this service, or you can make an appointment with a sports medicine center.

For the assessment, you will be asked to complete a health and medical questionnaire. This will identify any contraindi-cations such as a heart condition, pain during physical activity, dizziness, joint problems, drugs, pregnancy, and other factors that may influence your training routine.

Normal resting heart rate for adults is sixty to eighty beats per minute. Normal resting blood pressure in adults is 120/80 millimeters of mercury (systolic over diastolic BP). Day-to-day factors can influence these values, so it is best to measure more than once.

Body Measurements

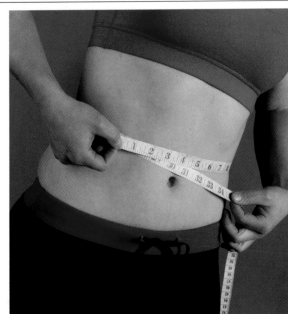

- Baseline girth measurements should include the right and left arms, right and left thighs (at the crotch), chest (under the armpits), waist, and hips (widest part).

- Body mass index (BMI) is a measure of body fat based on height and weight. A desirable ratio for women is 20.0 to 24.9.

Body-Fat Testing

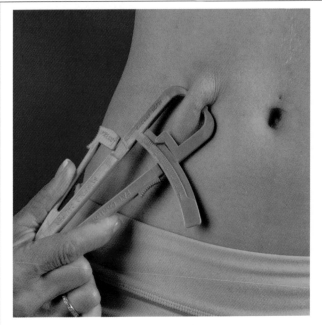

- Body composition is the ratio of fat to nonfat components of the body.

- A skin fold test is a measurement of subcutaneous fat.

- Weight training promotes the loss of unhealthy fat.

- Fat is located in other internal parts of the body and is necessary for healthy function.

A body-fat composition test is imperative to monitor fat loss and lean muscle gains. On your own you can perform a one-minute push-up and sit-up test, which will give you useful base values against which you can gauge your improvements.

The important points of these measurements are to understand your current fitness and health status, to formulate personal goals, and to track your progress. Repeat the fitness assessment every eight weeks if you are on a weight-loss program.

Forward Bend

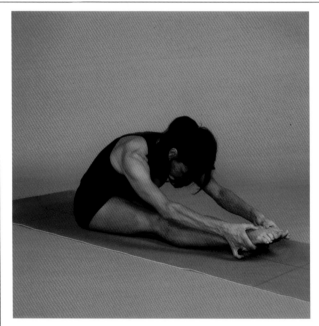

- *Flexibility* is defined as the ability of a joint to move freely through a full range of motion.

- Test your flexibility by sitting with your back, hips, and head against a wall and legs fully extended. Reach forward.

- Note how far you can go. Reassess every six to eight weeks

Goals

Goals are personal. Make your goals specific to your individual needs and desires. The best goals are those that involve a challenge, requiring you to reach beyond your comfort zone, yet are not entirely unattainable. Write them down, read them frequently, and visualize them happening. Believe that you can accomplish what you set out to do and don't let negative influences steer you off track.

For example:

- Lift weights Monday, Wednesday, and Friday before work.

- Elevate heart rate (sweat) on Tuesdays and Thursdays for 20 minutes.

PLANES OF MOTION, TERMINOLOGY

A functionally sound program should incorporate dynamic, multiplane movements into training

In order to learn the movements used in weight training, it is important to understand how they are described. It is not critical to memorize the details, but learning a few basic concepts will ensure that you are prepared for future references.

When performing even a simple motion like opening a door, your body performs a combination of movements in-volving three perpendicular planes. The planes describe motion relative to your body at a neutral stance.

The median plane, also called the sagittal plane, divides the body down the middle into left and right halves. Movement along this plane includes front to back movements like sit-ups and leg curls.

Human Anatomy

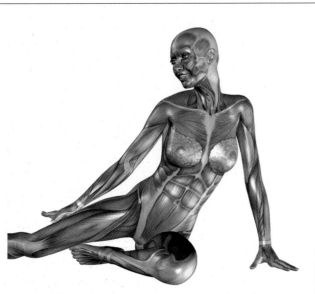

- There are six hundred skel-etal muscles in the human body.

- Complex movement and positions can be commu-nicated using planes to describe motion.

- Real-world movements are typically in all three planes.

- Both elbows above show a combination of extension, supination, and abduction in all three planes.

Median Plane

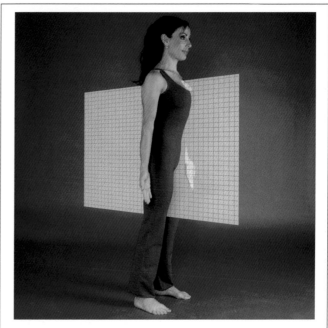

- Movement solely in the me-dian plane means that your body doesn't move across the plane.

- Sit-ups and your leg swing during walking are examples of movements in the median plane.

- Motion that is restricted to a single plane is called uniplanar motion.

The frontal plane, also called the coronal plane, divides the body into front and back halves. An example of movement along this plane is the motion of your arms and legs during jumping jacks.

The horizontal plane, also called the transverse plane, divides the body horizontally into upper and lower halves. Looking side to side and rotating at the waist are examples of motion in the horizontal plane.

ZOOM

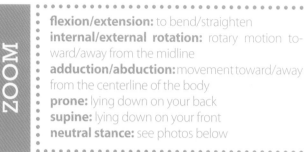

flexion/extension: to bend/straighten
internal/external rotation: rotary motion toward/away from the midline
adduction/abduction: movement toward/away from the centerline of the body
prone: lying down on your back
supine: lying down on your front
neutral stance: see photos below

Frontal Plane

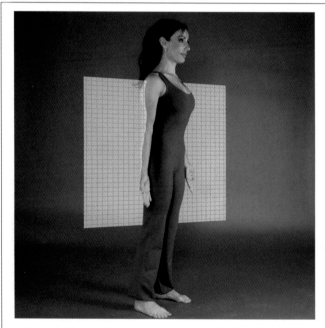

- Frontal plane movements include flexing your torso side to side and shrugging your shoulders.

- Lifting your arms out to the side would be an example of abduction—moving away from the body centerline—along the frontal plane.

Horizontal Plane

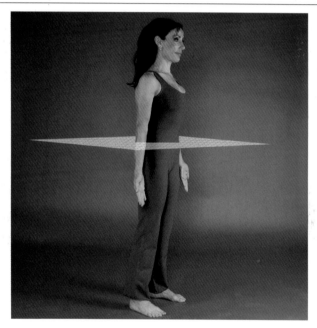

- Examples of horizontal planar movements include rotation of the elbow and knee and rotation of the head and torso.

- Another way to think about a plane of motion is that it includes all motions parallel to that plane.

13

FORM AND TECHNIQUE

Engaging your abdominals or pulling "navel to spine" is different from sucking in your stomach

Proper lifting always involves neutral body position. If your lifting form is off, even slightly, you risk injury and discomfort and compromise results. Neutral body position, neutral spine, good lifting form, and proper alignment will be referred to throughout this book. They incorporate the same tenets and apply to standing, lying, and seated positions.

In neutral body position, the head is high, neck long, chin centered, and shoulders down and retracted, not hunched. Imagine putting your shoulder blades in your back pocket. The spine is long, lean, and centered, maintaining its natural curve.

The abdominals are drawn in so that the rib cage is connected and the muscles around the spine are reinforced, like a corset.

Incorrect Chest Press Form

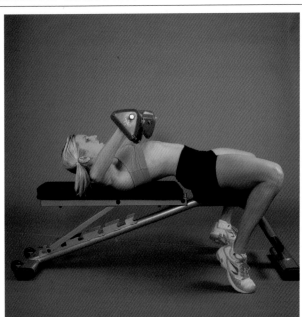

- Poor form can cause sprains, strains, tearing of the muscles, tendonitis, rotator cuff tears, nerve damage, and even fractures and dislocations.

- Bouncing weight off of your body, using momentum, changing a plane of motion, straining, tensing, protruding your abs, being in a hurry, not breathing, and overarching are all bad form.

Correct Chest Press Form

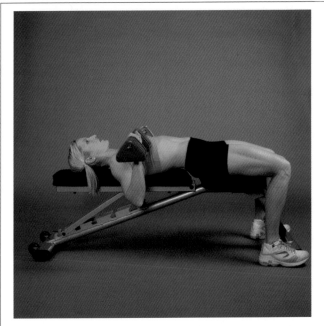

- Good form will maximize results and reduce injury.

- Avoid lifting too much weight or "cheating" (recruiting from other body parts, often resulting in straining).

- Move methodically and focus on the working muscles.

- EXHALE when PRESSING and INHALE when LOWERING weights.

Engage or scoop the innermost abdominals (transversus abdominis) by pulling the navel to the spine. This is different from sucking the stomach in, which causes you to hold your breath. Tuck the pelvis slightly, while maintaining length of the spine.

Hips and ankles align with the shoulders, while keeping the knees soft. Plant the feet evenly so that they bear an equal amount of weight. Avoid hyperextending or sinking into your joints. Neutral body position is not only important during your training but in the movements of everyday life.

LIFTING

Incorrect Squat Form

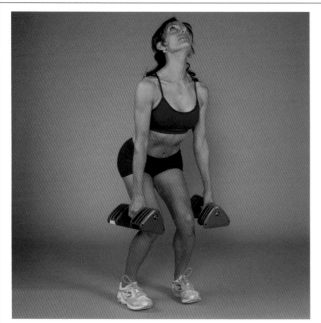

- STOP the movement if you cannot perform it properly.

- Poor form includes a swayed back, protruding abs, hunched shoulders, and an upward-thrusting neck.

- Knees collapsing to the center, or "bowing" out, during a squat is dangerous.

- Excessive weight on your toes will strain the knees.

Correct Squat Form

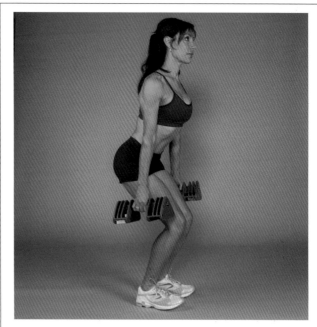

- Stand with weight evenly distributed, hips square, pelvis slightly tucked, shoulders down, and abs pulled in.

- Lower your body, keeping knees aligned with thighs and feet, and even weight on each foot.

- Squat until thighs are parallel with the floor, without extending knees beyond the toes.

FOCUS AND BREATH

Exhale through your mouth during hard efforts; inhale through your nose during the easy part

Breathing strengthens your respiratory and immune systems. It also reduces stress. A conscious breath can help you focus on the moment and center your body and mind.

Until you reach a level of proficiency in your fitness discipline, you may find that you concentrate so hard on your form and movement that you forget to breathe—or you breathe irregularly. Even more experienced athletes must resist the temptation to hold their breath when an exercise becomes particularly difficult. Holding your breath can cause light-headedness and increase blood pressure. In extreme cases, fainting, stroke, and heart attack may occur. This is not good for creating a good fitness experience!

Lotus Pose

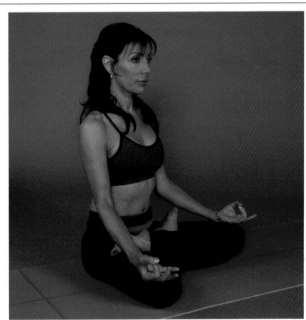

- Practice breathing in the Lotus Pose.

- Cross legs, placing equal weight on both sit bones.

- Lengthen spine and neck. Shoulders down, ears over shoulders, chin level to floor.

- Lift chest away from your navel. Create width across your collarbone. Soften your neck and face. Breathe slowly and concentrate.

Upright Big Toe Hold

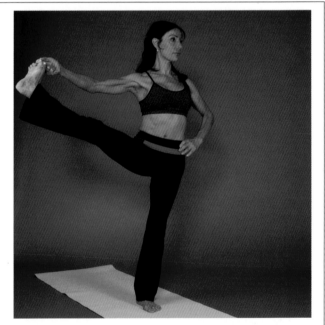

- Moves that incorporate balance train the body to breathe mindfully.

- Without deep breath, muscles will not receive sufficient oxygen and will therefore tighten.

- Breath should be natural, continuous, and not forced during activity.

- Focused breathing will help draw your mental energy to the task at hand.

The best way to breathe during weight lifting is to exhale during the contraction or concentric part of the exercise and inhale during the negative or eccentric part of the exercise. An easy way to think of these terms is that the contraction is the hard part, usually when you are lifting the weight and moving against gravity or some other resistance. Eccentric motion refers to the easy part, when you are bringing the weight back to starting position or moving with gravity. Remember to use this breathing rhythm for every exercise in this book!

ZOOM

Yoga and Pilates have taught us more about breath. The *Now* philosophy in Yoga claims we are allotted a certain number of breaths per lifetime. How we choose to illustrate that then becomes our practice of longevity. By improving fitness, you reduce your respiration rate, thereby improving your chances of breathing longer.

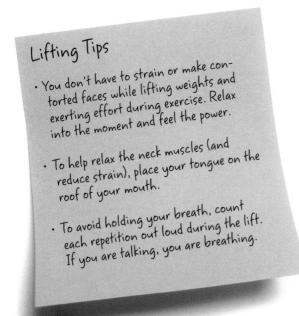

Lifting Tips

• You don't have to strain or make contorted faces while lifting weights and exerting effort during exercise. Relax into the moment and feel the power.

• To help relax the neck muscles (and reduce strain), place your tongue on the roof of your mouth.

• To avoid holding your breath, count each repetition out loud during the lift. If you are talking, you are breathing.

Focus

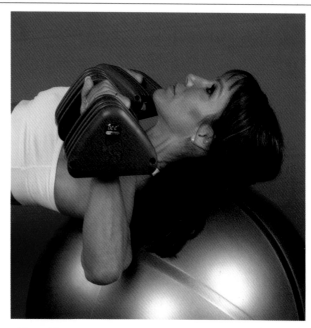

• Mental focus is an essential part of all sports.

• Centering the mind during weight lifting will help keep you in the moment, reducing anxiety and stress.

• A breathing technique to accomplish this is to inhale deeply through your nose and exhale slowly through your mouth.

17

WEIGHT, REPS, SETS

Learn the language of weight lifting and understand how to set up your personal program

There are three main variables to weight lifting: 1) how much weight is used; 2) how many repetitions or "reps" of the exercise are performed; and 3) how many sets are completed. One rep is equal to one completion of an exercise; for example, one biceps curl. A group of reps makes up a set; for example, a set of twelve biceps curls.

Another variable is the length of rest between sets. Typical weight-lifting practice for novice and intermediate fitness levels is to rest approximately 60 to 120 seconds between sets.

A final variable is how fast you perform one repetition. Aim for a smooth and controlled motion; avoid jerky movements.

Adjustable Dumbbells

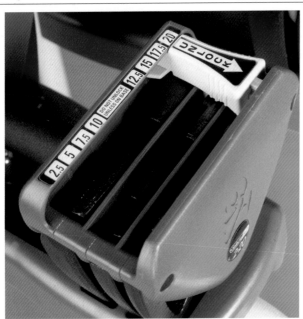

- Adjustable dumbbells provide multiple options in one piece of equipment. The weight range may be 2.5 to 20 pounds in 1.25-pound increments.

- They are compact, safe, convenient, and easy to adjust.

- Choose dumbbells with a comfortable and secure grip.

Repetition, Start Position

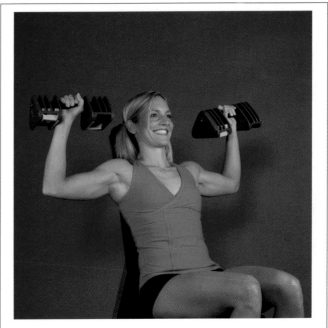

- One "rep" is a completion of an exercise from the starting position through the full contraction of the muscle to the finish position.

- The start position for an overhead press is weights at shoulder level, palms forward, hands firmly gripping the dumbbell, and body in proper lifting form.

A tempo count of two-zero-four is a good guideline. The lifting or concentric phase of the exercise should last for two counts. Pause momentarily; this represents the zero count. The returning or eccentric phase of the exercise should last four counts.

To increase muscular strength and power, aim for three to five sets of 6 to 8 reps per exercise using heavy weights. If you want to focus on muscular endurance and a slimmer body, perform three to five sets of 8 to 12 reps using weight that is an effort to lift.

Contrary to fat-buster methods of training, it is unnecessary to lift a weight for 20 to 25 reps. It can put you at risk for overtraining and is not recommended for long-term programs. Because of the potential for orthopedic injury in people 50 years and older, 10 to 15 reps may be more appropriate.

For the first 14 weeks of strength training, one set versus multiple sets of training will result in similar strength gains. After that, you must add variety to your routine every six to eight weeks.

Rest between Sets

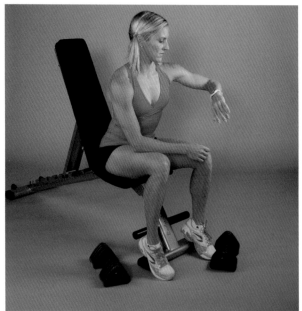

- A set is a group of repetitions of one exercise. A typical strength and endurance set involves 8 to 12 reps.

- After each set, place the weights on the floor and rest.

- When your allotted time for rest is complete (usually 60 to 120 seconds), start another set.

Full Range of Motion

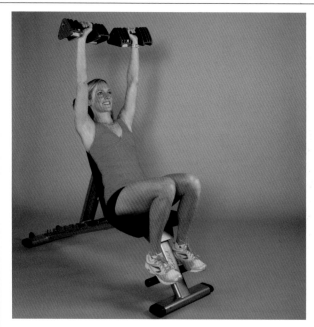

- Exercising to full range of motion allows muscles to develop completely.

- It allows muscles to stretch before contraction, increasing the number of muscle fibers being recruited, producing maximum results, and preventing injury.

- Typical household activities do not move your joints through a full range of motion.

PROGRAM BASICS

With limited time and resources, it is possible to fit in a quality workout—anywhere, anytime

Women respond well to a program that includes a twenty- to forty-minute weight-training routine at least three days per week and a twenty- to sixty-minute cardio session four to six days per week. Stretching and mind-body exercise should be incorporated into the program as well.

If you are so busy that you absolutely cannot block out this amount of time to train, choose a minimal daily plan. Something is always better than nothing. One or two body-weight exercises and/or stretching will keep you from getting too far off track.

A weight-training program that includes compound movements is a great way to get fit and manage time efficiently.

Defined Muscles

Muscles mature with age. Women who start an exercise program in their twenties will realize more defined musculature from repetitive use in their forties and beyond. Definition comes from the ability to contract the muscles harder and from staying lean. This explains why Madonna is more ripped today than she was early in her career.

Narrow Push-up

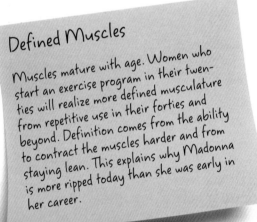

- Push-ups are an excellent exercise and can be done anywhere, anytime. Different hand placement will highlight different muscular focus.

- Beginners can start either against a wall or on knees to build strength and provide a fitness base.

- Performing hundreds of push-ups daily is not recommended. Your body needs time to repair itself.

Compound movements include exercises that work two or more muscle groups at a time (squats, lunges, step-ups). Exercising these large muscle groups burns more calories, too. And exercising the hips, buttocks, and thighs with minimal rest between sets will stimulate fat loss.

A superset is a training technique where you combine two exercises in a row with little rest in between. Supersets are perfect for busy women who want a challenge and intensity. Supersets can be demanding, so work your way up to this advanced routine.

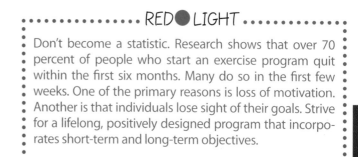
LIFTING

Overhead Press

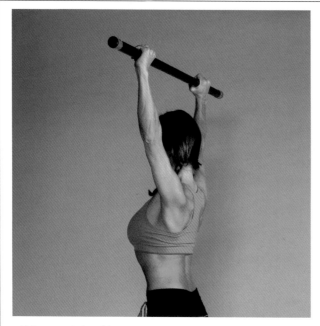

- Using a weighted bar or a barbell in your workout routine is an excellent addition to weight training.

- A standing overhead press demands core strength while working the shoul-ders, arms, and back muscles.

- Resistance training can take on many forms: Body weight is another example of resistance training.

Cycling

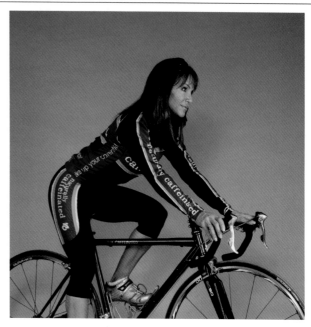

- Dedicate one day to a long, slow, distance training session, between one-and-a-half and three hours. Cycling, a non-weight-bearing activity, is easy on your body for this duration.

- Endurance is a must if you want to burn extra calories.

- Breaking from routine forces your body to adapt, getting stronger and fitter.

21

PLATE-LOADED MACHINES
Stacking your own weights on a machine and physically replacing them on racks is empowering

You can find plate-loaded weight-lifting machines in most fitness centers and gyms. They can be a bit bulky, so they tend to stand out. They use a weight plate that is manually placed, or racked, on a barbell for added resistance. The plates can weigh between 2.5 pounds and 45 pounds. The larger size requires full attention when loading and unload-

ing. A slip of the hand, so to speak, can lead to a potential toe-crushing moment.

Once racked, plate-loaded machines are safe to use and versatile. They are convenient for lifting and require less coordination than free weights. They are also biomechanically sound, meaning they are of good structure and function to the mechanics

Weight Plates

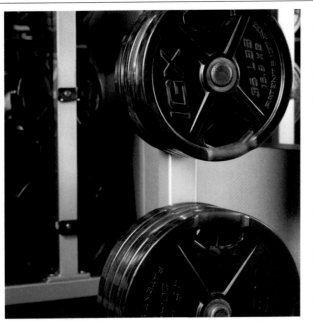

- Standard weight plates slip around the end of the barbell to add resistance to the equipment.

- Weight plates are stored on the sides of machines and on freestanding racks.

- Re-rack when you're done—that means put them away!

- Gym etiquette dictates sharing the machine with others between your sets if someone is waiting.

Leg Press

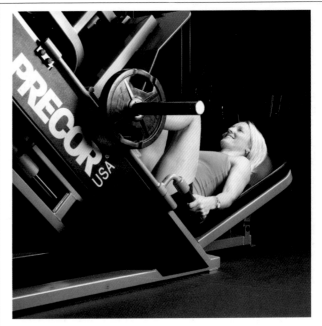

- Seated leg-press machines build lower-body power and muscular strength, complementing your training program.

- Add weight plates manually.

- Sit with proper lifting form. Place your feet shoulder-width apart and press the sled plate up and lower down to 90 degrees.

of the human body. Many plate-loaded machines can be used for a variety of exercises, targeting every body part. The Smith machine can be used for squats, which shape and strengthen the buttocks and legs. A bench can be placed under the bar for incline, decline, and flat upper body movements.

If you have never crawled into a plate-loaded machine, or placed your feet on the platform in preparation for a leg press, you have missed out on an incredibly powerful feeling. Learn to master a couple of these machines so that you can add variety and pure power to your training.

Smith Machine

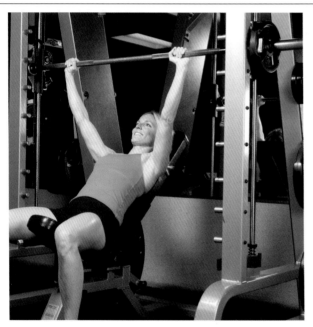

- Smith machines stabilize the motion of the exercise.

- Add weight plates and adjust the bench under the bar for chest press.

- Sit with neutral body position and press the bar up and down so it lands just above your breasts.

Seated Calf Raise

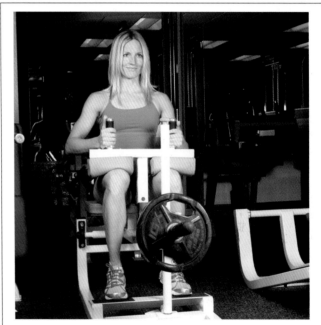

- The seated calf machine develops your calf muscles.

- Add weight plates.

- Sit with the knee pad on your thighs and adjust your body so the balls of your feet are on the foot platform with free heels.

- Raise your heels as high as possible, then lower them.

WEIGHT-STACK MACHINES

Imagine lying down, preparing for a set, and moving a pin to change resistance

Weight-stack machines are *selectorized,* meaning you select the weight. They are designed for one specific motion. You'll find a variety of different brands and styles to exercise every body part. To operate these machines, you simply need to make a couple adjustments on the machine, and never physically load a weight plate.

Changing the amount of weight is easy. A pin is used to designate your desired amount of resistance in increments of 5 to 10 pounds, depending on the machine. Until radical change happens, get comfortable with the standard pin/handle/knob styles. Consider these machines the "plug and play."

Weight-Stack Plates

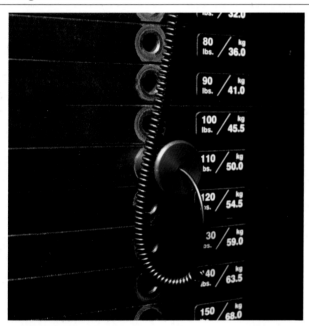

- Weight stacks allow the same machine to be used to provide several levels of resistance over the same range of motion.

- To change weight, place a pin into the slot.

- During movement, the plates above the pin are lifted and the plates below do not rise.

Reverse-Fly Machine

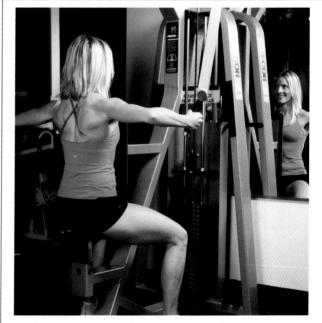

- Reverse-fly machines target the rear deltoids (back of the shoulders).

- Adjust the seat so the handles are even with shoulders. Face the machine and grab the handles.

- Pull the bar back as far as you can, pivoting from the shoulder joint and not the elbows.

- Stay in the same horizontal plane during movement.

Weight-stack machines are great for beginners because they require very little instruction. They also allow you to isolate muscle groups, which can be beneficial for body-specific training. A couple of examples of weight-stack machines that complement a free-weight program include the lying and seated leg curl, which targets the hamstrings, or the back of the legs; the leg-extension machine for the quads, or front of the legs; and the chest-fly and rear-delt, or back of shoulder exercises for the upper body and shoulders.

The downside of weight machines is that they do not recruit the small muscles. They follow a fixed range of motion that is not realistic in the real world of movement. If you want to focus on burning more calories and body fat, compound, balancing, and functional movement are your best choices.

Use weight machines when you are starting out and don't feel comfortable working out in the free-weight area or when you need to mix up your routine or target a particular muscle. If your motivation is lacking, selectorized machines provide a mentally easy training day. If you find your balance is off during menstruation, these machines are a great option.

Chest-Press Machine

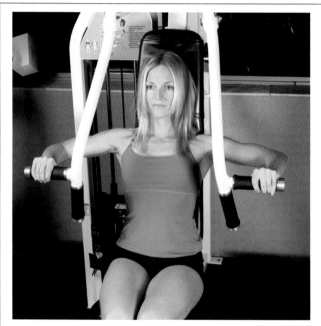

- Seated chest press is an upright version of the traditional lying or supine dumbbell or bar press.

- Adjust seat height. Sit with proper lifting form.

- Grasp the handles even with your chest and push the bars away from your body.

- Return to start with smooth controlled movement.

Seated Leg Extension Machine

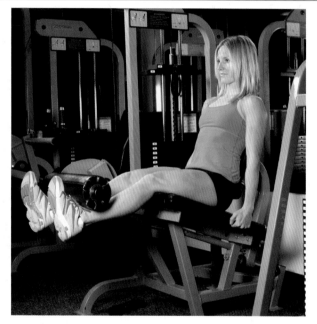

- Seated leg extensions define the quadriceps—the large thigh muscle on the front of the leg.

- Leg extensions are not recommended for individuals with knee injuries.

- Adjust seat so lower leg moves freely.

- Sit with good form. The machine arm should hit the front of your ankle.

- Extend your leg.

CABLE-MOTION SYSTEMS

A selection of handles near cable machines accommodates a variety of body-specific exercises

Cable-motion systems refer to any exercise with adjustable cables that allow your joints to move normally, freely, and painlessly through flexion and extension. This is referred to as a full range of motion. Cable-motion systems use weight stacks on one end connected to a pulley system on the other. There is a carabineer attachment for a handle, rope, or bar.

This is the part you pull, press, and move during exercise.

Picture an elastic-band exercise where you anchor the end of the band to a door and pull the cable for resistance. The tightness of the band is the resistance. The cable system is similar, only the cable does not stretch, so you lift the weight plate. You can move the cable in any direction and design a

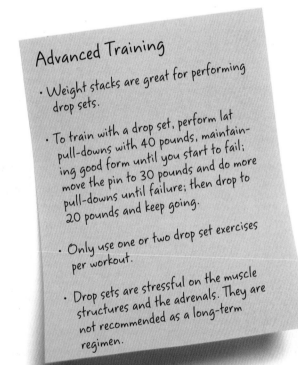

Advanced Training

- Weight stacks are great for performing drop sets.

- To train with a drop set, perform lat pull-downs with 40 pounds, maintaining good form until you start to fail; move the pin to 30 pounds and do more pull-downs until failure; then drop to 20 pounds and keep going.

- Only use one or two drop set exercises per workout.

- Drop sets are stressful on the muscle structures and the adrenals. They are not recommended as a long-term regimen.

FreeMotion Fitness Machine

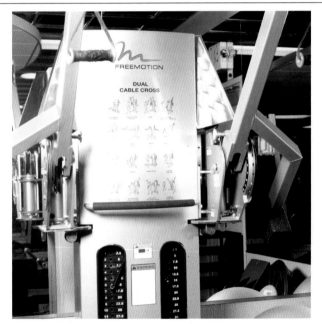

- FreeMotion Fitness machines are dual-cable cross machines capable of working the entire body through a full range of motion.

- Dual pulleys create smooth resistance.

- Multiple adjustments accommodate all sizes and fitness levels.

- Machines are compact and take up minimal space in a gym.

total-body program around this piece of equipment. A variety of handles provided at the gym are excellent tools to mix up your routine.

While plate-loaded and weight-stack machines limit the use of small, stabilizer muscles, cable systems effectively recruit them much like free weights do. In addition, cable systems provide a progressive resistance load; the amount of resistance increases throughout the range of motion. Progressive resistance is critical to developing strength.

Cable Crossover

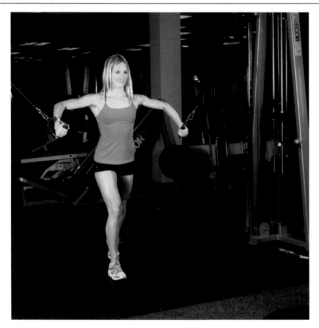

- Cable crossover machines take up a lot of space and are the centerpiece of most gyms.

- Stations provide a number of exercise options for every body part.

- Upper and lower pulleys provide smooth movement.

- Elastic toners (home equipment) can duplicate cable crossover exercises.

Lat Pull-Down

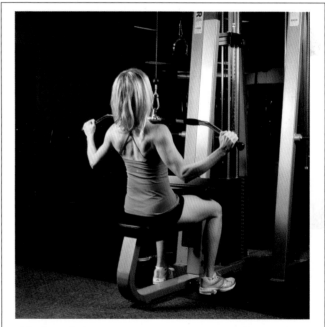

- The lat pull-down is a high fixed cable, typically connected to the cable crossover machine.

- It has a seat with roller pads to hold your legs down. A

- carabiner at the top allows different attachments.

- If you cannot do pull-ups, this exercise is a good alternative for training the same muscle group.

EQUIPMENT 101

27

BENCHES, BARBELLS, DUMBBELLS

Our daily tasks, like lifting objects in the home, are essentially free-weight training

Purists agree that free weights are the best tool for life-ready weight training because they allow you to exercise in a free range of motion in any *plane of motion*. Free weights recruit the primary and secondary muscles—the muscles that move your body parts—and the stabilizers—the muscles that hold your parts in place and prevent you from being damaged

while you're moving. The basic equipment associated with the term *free weights* are dumbbells, barbells, and benches.

Let's understand these terms and their tools. A bench is used for a variety of workouts and comes in flat, incline, and decline styles. Barbells are long bars with weight plates attached on the ends. The total weight of barbells may be fixed

Adjustable Bench

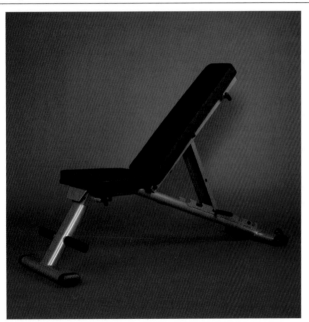

- Benches are used as a platform to sit or lie on or for stability when additional support is needed.

- Adjustable benches allow you to configure the height

- and angle, providing a variety of exercise options.

- Think *sturdy* when purchasing a bench.

Body Bars

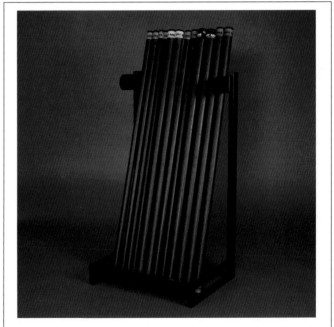

- Body Bars are solid steel fitness bars encased in rubber, making them easy to grip. They come in predetermined weight amounts with color-coded labels and can be used in place of traditional barbells.

- They are user-friendly and versatile.

- Because of their low-profile design, Body Bars can be incorporated into more types of workouts than traditional barbells.

due to permanently attached weights on each end or adjustable with the use of weight plates and a clasp to create your desired weight.

Traditional dumbbells that you will find in a gym come in two styles: a solid piece with hexagonal ends or a miniature version of a barbell with small weight plates held on with a bolt. Adjustable dumbbells are a third option, but they are more often found in a home gym than a commercial setting. The hex-dumbbells are the least comfortable to use because the end weight doesn't move, causing torque when you lift.

Dumbbells

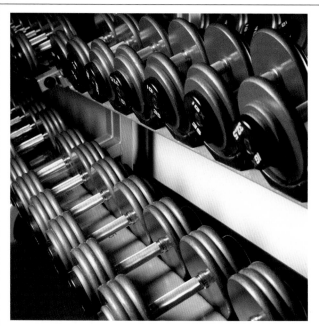

- Classic gym dumbbells are available in sizes from 5 pounds to 100 pounds in increments of 5 pounds.

- Stacked on a rack at the gym, they are convenient and accessible.

- Unlike many weight machines, dumbbells help develop balance and coordination, making them the best choice for functional strength training.

Barbells

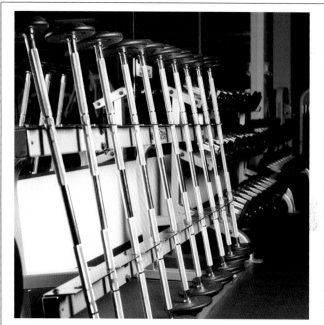

- Typical barbells have no torque because the ends rotate, making them comfortable to lift.

- In the gym, they are stored on a horizontal or vertical rack, making accessibility a main feature.

- It is not necessary to add weight to the bar itself.

FUNCTIONAL FITNESS TOOLS

What is the point of a workout if the program and exercises lack practical value?

According to both the American College of Sports Medicine and the American Council on Exercise, functional fitness is one of the biggest exercise trends. Functional fitness trains you to be prepared for life. Think of what you do every day—from lifting groceries and suitcases, to reaching over the counter, to running up and down stairs—all these movements require your body to respond in a nonlinear, dynamic fashion.

Functional fitness is core to our life-training program. It involves free weights, body-weight exercises that involve compound exercises, or the multi-joint movements that work several muscles or muscle groups at one time. Functional fitness tools look similar to children's playroom equipment, and

Stability Balls

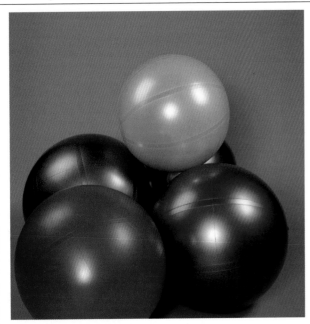

- Balance or stability balls develop balance, agility, strength, and proprioception.

  Less than 5'2" = 45cm ball
  5'2" to 5'8" = 55cm ball
  5'9" to 6'2" = 65cm ball
  6'3" to 6'9" = 75cm ball

- The correct size, based on your height, is a critical consideration.

Functional Fitness Equipment

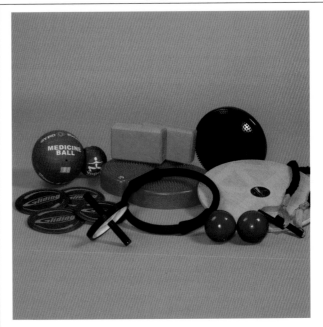

- Wobble boards, medicine balls, yoga blocks, elastic toners, Kettlebells (not shown), stability discs (or pillows), and Gliding discs are functional tools.

- Each piece of equipment adds variety and specificity to your training routine.

- Experiment with different products at a gym before purchasing.

for a good reason. They are designed to develop your mind and body. It is called **fun**ctional fitness because this category of exercise is designed to improve balance and agility, strengthen the stabilizer muscles needed for healthy movement, and increase proprioception in addition to increasing overall strength.

Whatever is impairing your ability to move comfortably—an existing injury, chronic conditions, joint problems, arthritis, lack of conditioning, or overtraining concerns—functional fitness can help.

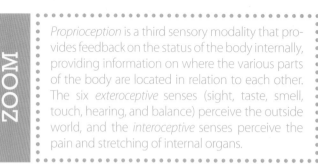

Proprioception is a third sensory modality that provides feedback on the status of the body internally, providing information on where the various parts of the body are located in relation to each other. The six *exteroceptive* senses (sight, taste, smell, touch, hearing, and balance) perceive the outside world, and the *interoceptive* senses perceive the pain and stretching of internal organs.

BOSU

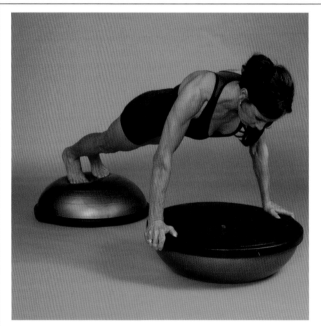

- BOSU is an acronym for "both sides up."

- The BOSU balance trainer is an inflated thick rubber dome on a flat, 25-inch round platform.

- It provides a total body workout with aerobic and strength routines and stretching, flexibility, and balance training.

Step Platform

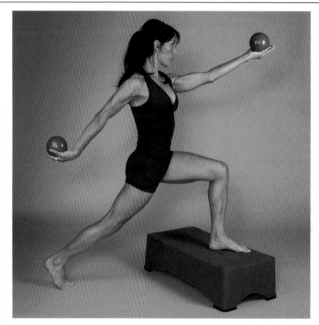

- A step can be used for cardio, strength, agility, and balance moves.

- Combined with other tools, a step provides unlimited fitness options.

- Plyometrics, which involve jumping, bounding, and hopping exercises, can be done on a sturdy step.

MUST-HAVE HOME EQUIPMENT

The outstanding selection of quality home fitness products makes purchasing yours easy and affordable

The major advantage of home equipment is convenience. You need a bulletproof system to keep your fitness focus at all times. Home equipment is the no-wait, squeeze-in-a-workout-twenty-four-hours-a-day, listen-to-your-own-music-as-loudly-as-you-want inspiration.

A treadmill or cardio machine at home is a fitness savior during bad weather. Knowing you don't have to drive or miss a scheduled workout is worth every dollar spent. You can shop online, through shopping channels or reliable used equipment sources, and find amazing deals and payment plans for your complete setup.

Minimally speaking, you should have: a piece of cardio

Yoga Mat and Elastic Toners

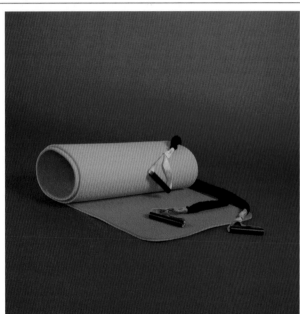

Bench and Stability Ball

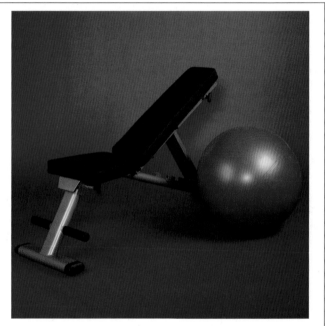

- Sleeved elastic toners are inexpensive, portable, and provide a total body training system. Look for a set that includes several levels of resistance and a door anchor attachment.

- Yoga mats come in man-made materials or natural fibers.

- Choose a durable mat that cleans easily and provides cushioning.

- Own a stability ball and a bench for maximum fitness benefits.

- Choose an adjustable bench that is sturdy and has incline, decline, and flat positions.

- Purchase a ball that is durable, will maintain its shape, and has eight panels that provide reinforcement.

- Balls that deflate easily are worthless for performing exercises.

equipment; something for resistance training; and stretching tools. The success of a home gym depends on your own motivation and having the right equipment that is easy to use and dependable and allows some variety.

A balanced training plan requires that you couple your home equipment practice with the outdoor world. Leaving the comfort of your home gym can take your fitness to another level. A training partner or social networking group will keep you motivated and on track when you need it most.

MAKE IT EASY

Home equipment should be durable and require little upkeep and repair. Cheap cardio products can be unstable, noisy, and hard on your joints. Shop from sources that have an unconditional return policy and customer service help lines. Set up your product according to dealer specifications. Use your machine as much as possible during the first two weeks.

Set of Adjustable Dumbbells

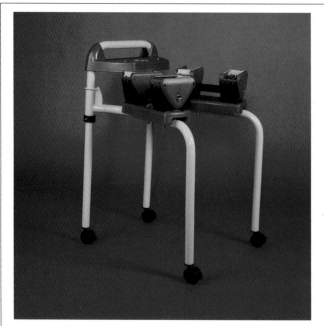

- Adjustable dumbbells are the best choice for home use.

- A simple quick lever instantly changes the SelectaBell dumbbell weight from 2.5 to 20 pounds, giving you control to make 1.25-pound incremental changes.

- Select a brand that comes with a stand and has wheels for portability.

Cardio Equipment

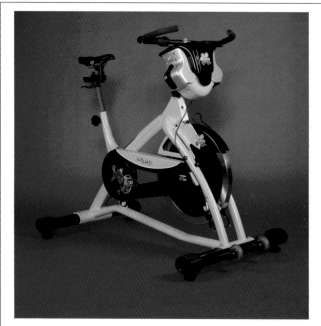

- A treadmill, elliptical trainer, or stationary bike is a must for cardiovascular training.

- Prepare to pay for good quality.

- Focus on the "guts" of the machine, more than superfluous bells and whistles.

- Stationary bikes should change resistance easily and pedal smoothly.

ONE-MINUTE WARM-UP

Can you distinguish between a warm-up and exercise if they both involve stretching or moving?

Let's agree to agree. A one-minute warm-up holds no credibility in the sports-training world. A one-minute warm-up, however, is still better than no warm-up. Warm-ups are recommended for a reason. They decrease the potential for injury and increase performance.

The intent of a warm-up is to increase blood flow to your working muscles by facilitating oxygenation and reducing fatigue. Muscle and connective tissue become more elastic and pliable, thus reducing their potential to tear.

Aerobic activity and stretching exercises are the principle forms of warm-ups recommended by professional trainers. A cardio warm-up, such as cycling, jumping jacks, or stepping

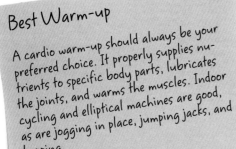

Best Warm-up

A cardio warm-up should always be your preferred choice. It properly supplies nutrients to specific body parts, lubricates the joints, and warms the muscles. Indoor cycling and elliptical machines are good, as are jogging in place, jumping jacks, and hopping.

Stretching a cold muscle can cause injury. If you do use stretching and a one-minute warm-up option, move gently, being careful not to strain.

Overhead Reach

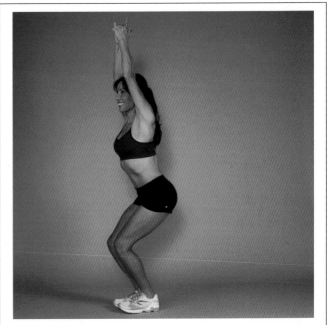

- Compound movements will increase your heart rate, supplying blood to the muscles.

- Squatting engages the large muscle groups.

- Reaching overhead creates another level of difficulty, helping the body warm up.

- Add a greater challenge by standing on one leg for thirty seconds.

in place, is better than stretching, because stretching a cold muscle can cause a tear or decrease strength. Choose a cardio warm-up as your priority option.

If you can't muster the energy for a cardio warm-up, then use compound stretching as a secondary plan. Compound stretches, where you engage your large muscles, will get your heart pumping faster than static stretches. You may ask, "At what point during my squat exercise warm-up am I just getting warm or actually exercising?" They both look similar on paper. If it makes more sense, consider sitting in a hot tub or taking a warm shower before exercise. These are both acceptable forms of a warm-up and easier to understand than moving to get you ready to move!

Develop your own conscience when it comes to the one-minute warm-up scenario. If you're so busy that this is the only option, then practice good aerobic warm-up form by not putting your knees or joints in a compromising position. If your choice is a compound stretch, temper your desire to do the splits or out-perform Gumby.

Forward Bend

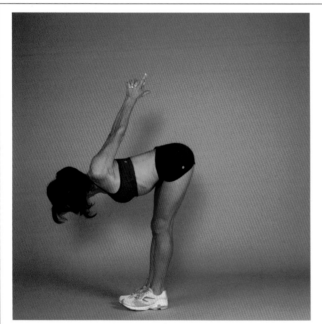

- The objective of moving and bending is not to stretch, but to get the heart pumping and oxygenate the muscles.

- Forward bending demands that your body stabilize and balance itself, which is another way of increasing your heart rate.

- Avoid overstretching during a warm-up.

Standing One-Leg Hold

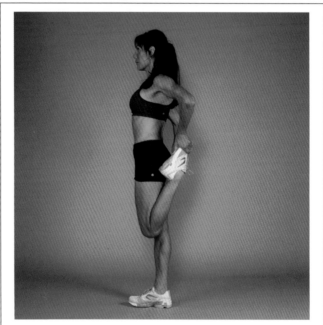

- Balancing on one foot creates a challenge for the body.

- Make sure to stabilize your core by pulling your belly to your spine.

- When grabbing the lifted foot behind you, gently counter-press during the movement by pressing away from your hand using your leg strength.

TOP CARDIO BLASTS
Getting the heart pumping is physiologically ideal, and it can mentally snap you into focus

Let's refresh our cardio knowledge. Cardio involves the circulatory system: heart, lungs, arteries, veins, and capillaries. A working muscle will burn energy, causing blood temperature to rise and the heart to beat faster. Once the heart rate increases, the blood vessels dilate, causing more blood and oxygen to be transported to the muscles, making them more

elastic and ready for the demands of exercise.

A sufficient cardio warm-up lasts ten minutes. Gym cardio machines are an excellent resource. You can easily monitor exactly how fast you're going and keep track of your time. Another option is a brisk walk or jog on your way to the gym!

The more fit you become, the easier it is to handle a lon-

Step-up Start

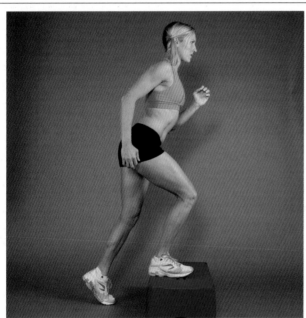

- Use a step for this step-up/step-down ten-minute warm-up.

- Start slowly, step onto the platform with your right foot, followed by your left foot.

- Step down with your left foot, followed by your right foot.

- Step up with your left and follow with your right.

- Repeat this sequence.

Step-up Finish

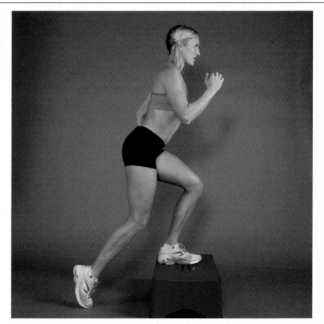

- Increase the tempo of your steps after a couple of minutes.

- Notice your heart rate increase. This is normal and expected.

- Stay light on your feet. Try not to pound or land flat-footed.

- You will feel less impact when you land by focusing on the up movement.

ger warm-up. Women who are endurance trained consider a long run or an hour-long cardio challenge a perfectly acceptable warm-up before engaging in strength training. This warm-up/double workout is a calorie-burning bonus! If you have got the time and the fitness, try upping your cardio warm-up to more than a ten-minute obligatory routine.

If there is no equipment to use for a cardio warm-up, fear not. Rapid step-ups and side lunges accomplish the task. After ten minutes, you should experience an increased heart rate, a light perspiration, and a healthy glow.

Side Lunge Start

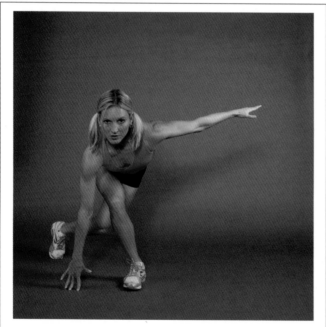

Side Lunge Finish

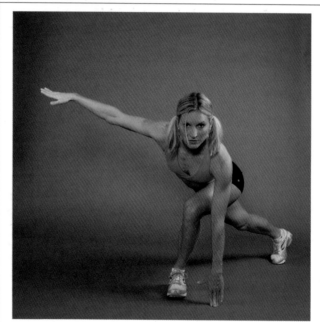

- A side lunge is a form of cardio warm-up.

- Facing forward, step right foot to side, keeping upper body stable and head up.

- Cross left leg behind body

and squat by slightly bending the right knee, keeping your weight on your right heel.

- Extend left arm out to the side and tap right hand to floor.

- Keeping your body forward and torso straight, repeat sequence on other side.

- Start by standing and stepping to side with left leg.

- Right leg sweeps behind the planted (left) foot, extending behind.

- Drop your left hand down, tap the floor, and extend your right arm to the side.

TOWEL STRETCHES

Towels create a pleasurable stretching experience, minimizing the challenges of limited flexibility

In a perfect world, you'd have a personal trainer or massage therapist help you stretch after a workout. This would be a form of stretching called *passive* stretching. It involves having another person move your body into stretches for you. The benefit is that you can usually stretch farther than on your own, lengthening the muscles, helping them relax, and increasing blood flow to remove waste products. Plus, it feels good to be pampered!

If an on-call stretching assistant is not an option, try a towel for some *active* stretching. Active stretching is when you put your body into positions that facilitate the lengthening of specific muscles or muscle groups. A towel's maneuverability

Overhead Towel Stretch

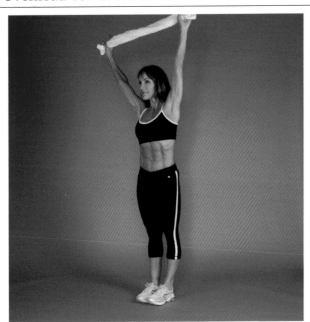

- Roll up a towel and grab both ends.

- Lift overhead with feet planted firmly.

- Pull energetically on both ends of the towel.

- Hold the towel up and keep pulling out for thirty to sixty seconds.

- Start circling the upper body in a rotational dynamic stretch.

Behind Back Towel Stretch

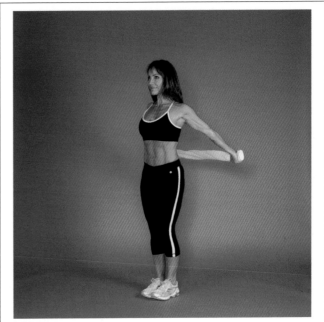

- Stretches chest, shoulders, and arms.

- Grab rolled-up towel with both hands behind your back.

- Pull energetically on both ends of the towel.

- Lift upward and hold for thirty to sixty seconds.

- If able, move from behind the back, overhead, and down the front of your body.

can assist getting to those difficult-to-stretch spots on your own. Towels are readily available when traveling, at home, and in the club. Depending on your level of flexibility, a small hand towel or larger bath towel will accommodate most individuals.

How long should you stretch? Recommended time is between thirty to sixty seconds per stretch. If it feels good, stretch longer. You can stretch every day, too. Just remember not to overstretch.

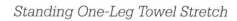

YELLOW ● LIGHT

Symptoms and signs of overstretching include tenderness and pain, bruising, inflammation, swelling, inability to move a joint or limb, or instability. A pull or tear of a muscle or tendon—the cord of tissue connecting the muscle to the bone—is usually a result of overstretching.

Hamstring Towel Stretch

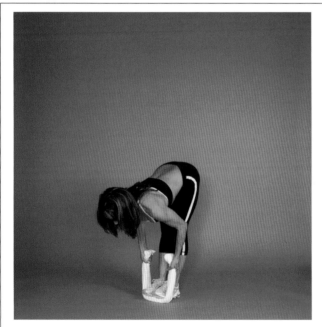

- Place rolled-up towel under your feet. Grab each end of the towel.

- Straighten your legs and bend forward with your back flat, bending at your hips only.

- Pull up on the towel to facilitate the stretch. Hold for thirty to sixty seconds.

- Try rounding your back for a lower-, middle-, and upper-back and spine stretch.

Standing One-Leg Towel Stretch

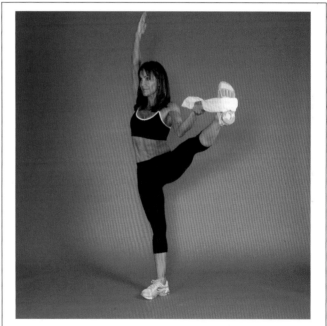

- Stretches the groin.

- Place rolled-up towel under one foot. Grab the ends of the towel in one hand.

- Lift your leg up to the front of your body, balancing on the standing leg. Hold for thirty to sixty seconds.

- Move your leg out to the side of the body. Hold for thirty to sixty seconds.

- Repeat on other side.

UPPER-BODY STRETCHES

Stretching is a form of preventive medicine; it reduces stress, improves flexibility, and aids recovery

Your face, neck, shoulders, upper back, chest, triceps, biceps, forearms, hands, and fingers fall into the category of upper-body parts for this section. You should stretch at the conclusion of a cardio or weight-training session. After an upper-body workout, stretching will help your muscles to maintain their proper length.

Strength conditioning causes the muscles to contract repeatedly, meaning they shorten in length. Failure to stretch sets you up for chronic muscle tightness. Muscle tightness and imbalance in the body's alignment is a vicious cycle.

If the muscles just below your neck, called the trapezius, are tight, chances are you are craning your head forward. Having

Upper-Neck/Trap Stretch

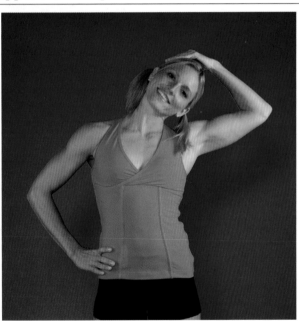

- Take one hand and place it on your hip or let it hang down the side of your body, palm in.

- Grasp your head with the other hand.

- Gently pull your ear toward your shoulder. Hold for thirty to sixty seconds.

- Repeat on other side.

Anterior Shoulder Stretch

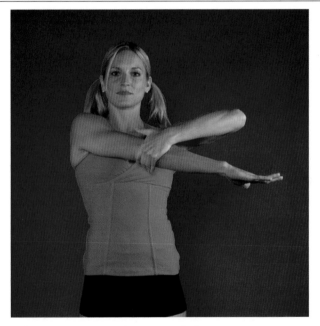

- Place one arm across the front of your body, palm down.

- Grasp your elbow with the other hand.

- Pull your arm across your body, keeping your torso straight. Hold for thirty to sixty seconds.

- Repeat on the other side.

your head forward puts your spine in a compromising position and will cause potential back pain. The lack of proper alignment can then create a chain reaction throughout the rest of your body. Bottom line: Don't skip a stretching session after lifting weights or exercising.

It might make sense to stop a workout a few minutes early so that you can spend more time on your stretching. This will start your recovery process immediately.

Note: The stretches in this section do not cover every upper-body part. Consult additional resources for more options and variations.

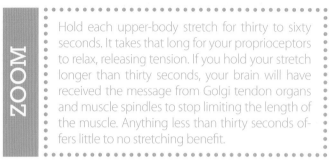
One-Arm Chest Stretch

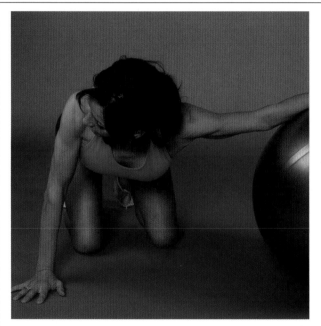

- Use a stability ball or any elevated surface.

- Kneel with the ball at your side. Place your arm on the ball at a 90 degree angle to the floor.

- Lower your chest and shoulder toward the floor, keeping your torso parallel with the floor.

- Hold for thirty to sixty seconds. Repeat on the other side.

Upper-Back Stretch

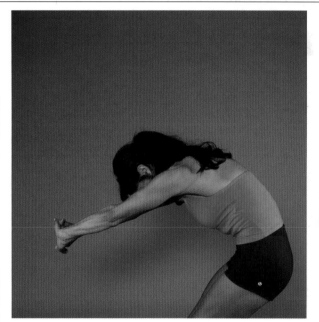

- From a standing position, clasp your hands in front of you, palms forward (internally rotating the arms).

- Drop into a three-quarters squat, legs together, abdominals engaged.

- Reach the hands away from your body while rounding your back.

- Hold for thirty to sixty seconds.

MID-BODY STRETCHES
Stretching is best done when warm because your muscles and tendons are more compliant

Your abdominals, middle and lower back, hips, and derrière comprise your mid-body for this section. Let's start by addressing the hips. The hips are the merging point of the lower and upper body. Hips respond to regular, gentle stretching, not sporadic force.

The abdomen is often overlooked when stretching. Stretch-

ing the abdominals can help massage your abdominal organs, relieve constipation, and improve blood flow to your brain. However, avoid stretching this area if you have a hernia, have had surgery, or are pregnant and past your second trimester.

The *gluteus maximus, medius, and minimus muscles* (glutes for short) make up the buttocks. This muscle group tightens

Bow Pose

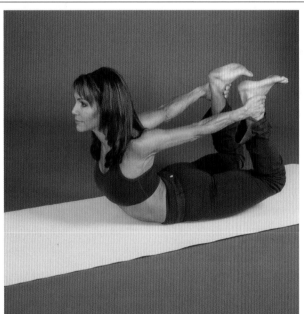

- Extends the spine, expands the chest, relieves respiratory problems, and strengthens the abdomen.

- Lie on your belly, arms by your sides. Bend your knees and grab your ankles.

- Lift your thighs and torso off the mat. Lengthen from your head, keeping your shoulders down.

- Hold for thirty seconds.

Cat Stretch

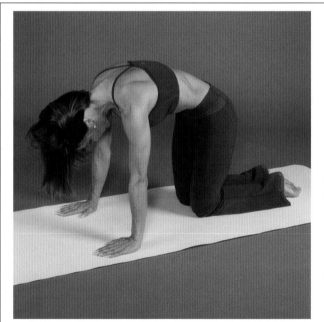

- Helps with flexibility of spine, neck, and shoulders. Helpful for menstrual cramps.

- On hands and knees, keep arms straight, fingers forward.

- Raise your head toward the ceiling, arching your spine and creating a concave back.

- Then lower your head, rounding your spine upward and pulling abdomen inward.

the more you sit and squat. It takes a certain amount of commitment and courage to move into poses that target the glutes. Getting past that point of discomfort is worth your while. Additional benefits of opening the hips and stretching the glutes and abdomen include a release of unwanted stress and a calming of the nervous system. You will feel grounded and relaxed after practicing these mid-body stretches.

Note: The exercises in this section do not cover every mid-body part you should stretch. Consult additional resources for more options and variations.

Pigeon Pose

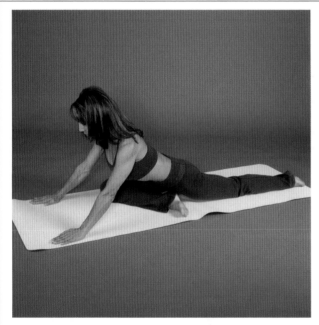

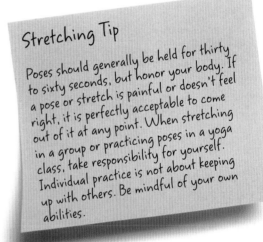

Stretching Tip

Poses should generally be held for thirty to sixty seconds, but honor your body. If a pose or stretch is painful or doesn't feel right, it is perfectly acceptable to come out of it at any point. When stretching in a group or practicing poses in a yoga class, take responsibility for yourself. Individual practice is not about keeping up with others. Be mindful of your own abilities.

- Revitalizes internal organs, stretches the thighs, hips, and groin.

- Hands flat on the floor, fingers forward.

- Bend your right leg, bringing your knee to the inside of your right hand.

- Extend left leg behind, grounding thigh to the floor and sink your pelvis downward. Fold forward.

LOWER-BODY STRETCHES

Static stretching relaxes the body; dynamic stretching, like mobility drills, prepares the body for activity

Your groin, quadriceps, hamstrings, knees, lower legs, calves, ankles, and feet comprise the lower body for this section. A pulled hamstring and groin tear are painful injuries. Either will put a stop to your training program for weeks if not months.

If you have chronically tight muscles, you may want to dedicate two parts of your training session to stretching. This can be accomplished after the warm-up before working out, and again after your workout. Learn to keep your lower body limber and loose. It helps with injury prevention and performance.

Let's spend a moment on your knees. If you suffer from knee pain, it may be due to weakness of connective tissue or tightness in other parts of the leg. Specific stretching exercises to

Groin Stretch

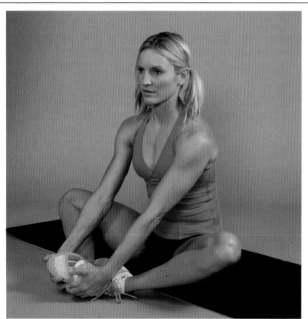

- With your knees bent, place the bottoms of your feet together in a seated position.

- Gently press the tops of the knees down with the elbows and lean forward.

- Hold thirty to sixty seconds.

- Variation: On hands and knees, abduct (widen) knees and lean forward.

Stability Ball Quad Stretch

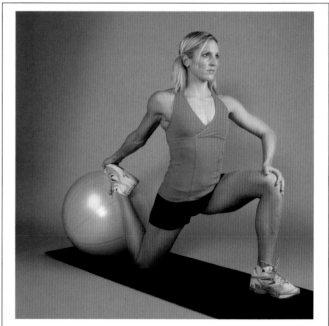

- Place the top of your right foot on top of the stability ball.

- Kneel with your left leg in a 90 degree position. Left leg is supporting your weight.

- Rise upward with your torso. Tuck your pelvis to increase the stretch.

- Hold thirty to sixty seconds.

help this area include stretching the calf, quads, and illiotibial (IT) track. The IT band connects the hip to the knee and can cause tightness and imbalance. Cyclists and runners know this tightness all too well. Adductor, or inner thigh, tightness can also contribute to knee pain, as it pulls the knee joint and the leg toward the inside. Any deviation in knee alignment can cause issues.

Note: The exercises in this section do not cover every lower-body part you should stretch. Consult additional resources for more options and variations.

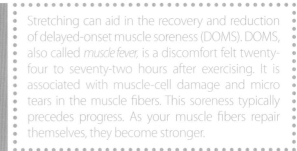
Forward Bend Stretch

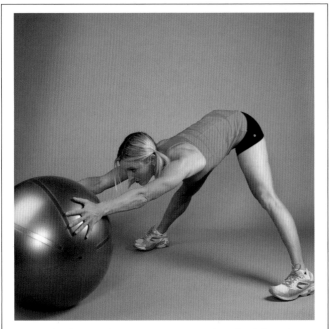

- Stretches legs and upper body.

- In a wide stance, place both hands on top of the ball.

- Keep your upper body and torso parallel to floor.

- Straighten both legs. Put your weight on your heels.

- Reach forward and continue dropping your chest.

- Hold thirty to sixty seconds.

Lateral Side Stretch

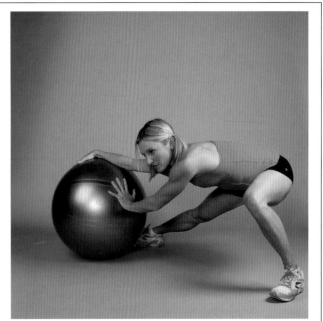

- In a forward bend position, roll the ball to your right side.

- Keep both hands on the ball.

- Lunge your leg opposite to the ball, bend knee to 90 degrees.

- Hold thirty to sixty seconds.

- Visualize your muscles extending as you stretch (think traction).

WARM-UPS, STRETCHES

TRANSVERSUS ABDOMINIS

When the transversus abdominis muscles contract, the waist narrows and the lower abdomen flattens

The term *six pack* is a common description of a ripped midsection. Chances are, you won't hear someone yell, "Nice transverse abdominals!" Yet, without this abdominal muscle being strong and trained, it's doubtful you'll hear any comments at all. Training with crunches alone will not give you a flat belly. Transversus abdominis exercises will.

The transversus abdominis (TVA) is the deepest of the abdominal muscles. The TVA wraps around the abdomen between the lower ribs and the top of the pelvis, connecting to the middle of the body.

The TVA muscles run laterally from the sides to the front, or anterior, of the body. The fibers run horizontally, which is why

Core Muscles

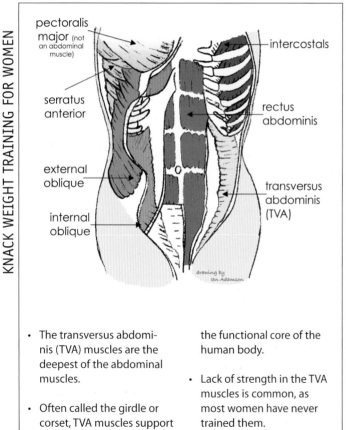

pectoralis major (not an abdominal muscle)

intercostals

serratus anterior

rectus abdominis

external oblique

transversus abdominis (TVA)

internal oblique

drawing by Ian Adamson

Incorrect Stability Form

Low back arch (space) and protruding rib cage indicate poor transversus abdominis strength.

- The transversus abdominis (TVA) muscles are the deepest of the abdominal muscles.

- Often called the girdle or corset, TVA muscles support

- the functional core of the human body.

- Lack of strength in the TVA muscles is common, as most women have never trained them.

- To target the transversus abdominis (TVA) muscles, a perfect balance of compression and stabilization in the low back must be maintained.

- If the low back arches up, you are NOT engaging your TVA muscles.

- Bad form includes poor neck and head alignment and the rib cage popping out.

they are called *transversus*. They connect to the diaphragm, helping with inhalation. The TVA muscles are stabilizers for the individual spinal segments. They help create space between vertebrae and assist posture. They compress the ribs and help pregnant women deliver their children.

The TVA muscles activate before any strong movement takes place in your body. Lack of strength in the TVA muscles can lead to back pain, injury, and disappointment in achieving your fitness goals.

Correct Stability Form

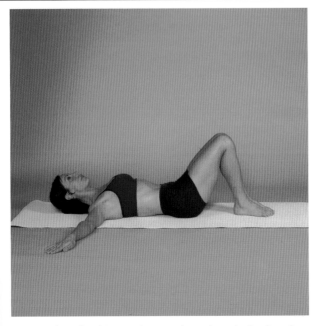

- Proper form for this exercise will be the standard for all movements.

- Lie on your back with the spine energetically pressed to floor.

- Lengthen the back and neck, chin centered, shoulders retracted.

- Tuck the pelvis slightly, rib cage pulled in. Draw the belly button in toward the spine.

One-Leg Stability Activation

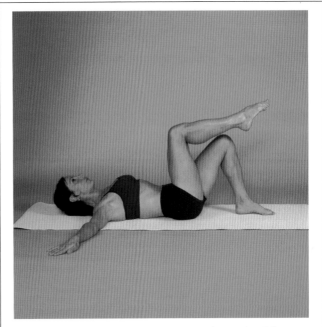

- To activate the TVA muscles, raise one foot off the floor and do not change the position of the body. Concentrate on pressing the low back energetically into the floor.

- Keep the angle of the lifted leg, bent knee equal throughout the lift.

- Do not extend the knee past 90 degrees.

CORE CONDITIONING

47

STABILITY CRUNCH

Instability can cause excessive stiffening of the muscles, and the joints will lock to compensate

Using a stability ball in your fitness program will help you develop greater core strength through the rectus abdominis. This is the long, flat abdominal muscle located on either side of the torso that creates the washboard look.

Stability balls allow your body to break a horizontal plane—a limiting factor when doing floor crunches—allowing you to work a greater range of motion. The more range you can achieve in a ball crunch, the more fibers you will recruit, ultimately achieving greater strength and better results.

Performing abdominal exercises on a stability ball will also improve your balance and coordination and is good for agility and conditioning.

Stability Ball Crunch Start

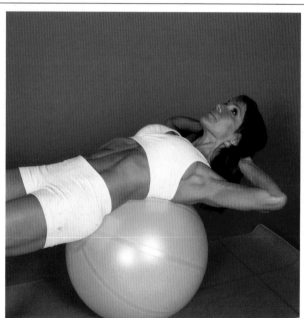

- Sit on the ball. Walk your feet forward until your hips are off the ball and your back is resting on it.

- Place your feet shoulder-width apart for additional balance.

- Gently place both hands behind your head, keeping your elbows wide.

- Gently press head into hands if you feel neck strain.

Stability Ball Crunch Finish

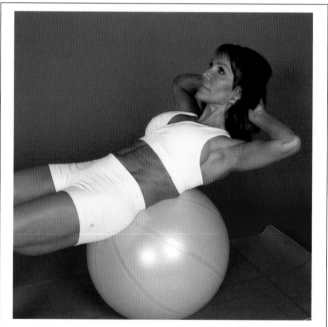

- Without moving the ball or dropping your hips, curl your upper body toward the ceiling.

- Keep your head neutral with space between chin and chest.

- Keep constant tension throughout the crunch. You should feel a burn.

- Change your arm and body position for variations.

Ball crunches can be done from a variety of angles. Small changes to your arms, legs, and where the ball sits under your body will create less or more resistance. To add challenge to your stability ball crunch routine, try an approach similar to pyramid training.

Once you are comfortable with the crunching motion, play with different hand/arm positions in the same set of repetitions. Options include over your chest for 10 reps, behind your head for 10, stretched out behind you for 10, one elbow up at a time for 10, and then reverse the process.

Reverse Crunch Start

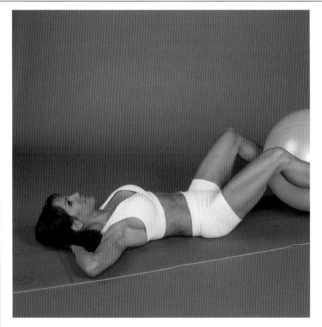

- Beginners may find this position challenging.

- Lie on your back and place the stability ball between your feet.

- Engage your transversus abdominis muscles by pressing your lower back to the floor. Place your hands behind your head.

Reverse Crunch Finish

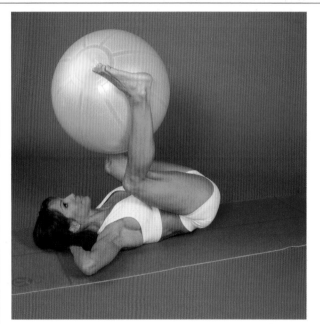

- Contract your abs by lifting your feet off the floor (keeping the ball squeezed between your legs).

- Avoid arching your back or deviating from proper form.

- To increase the difficulty, lift your chest slightly toward the ball.

- This exercise may cause low back strain. Stop if you feel discomfort.

CORE CONDITIONING

LEG RAISE

Leg raises, a form of abdominal training, work the abdominals and hip flexors simultaneously

It's probably a good time to state that technical literature and studies of abdominal training do not distinguish between individual exercises for the top half and lower half of the rectus abdominis and obliques.

Any effective exercise for your abdominals will recruit a combination of core muscles. We do know that the trans-

versus abdominis muscles need individual attention and can be targeted by specific exercises. Even so, you will still recruit other core muscles in the process.

Leg raises are excellent to work the superficial abdominals and the hip flexors. The hip flexors include the Iliacus and the Psoas major, the muscles that bend the hip. The abdominals

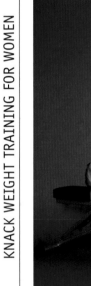

Straight Leg Raise Start

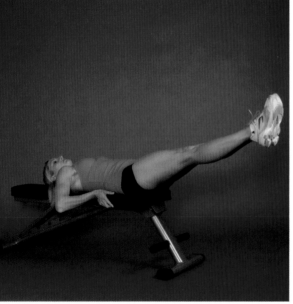

- Lie on your back, with legs off the end of a flat bench.

- Place your hands on the side of the bench near your torso. Keep legs parallel with the floor.

- Head should be relaxed and resting on the bench.

Straight Leg Raise Finish

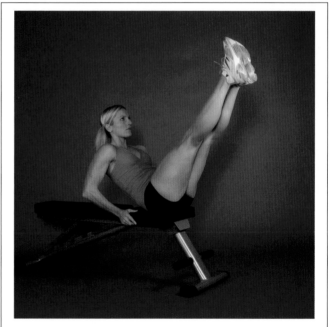

- Keeping your legs as straight as possible, raise them into the air while lifting your upper body.

- Aim for a V position.

- Concentrate on using your abdominals for the workload, not your legs.

- Use your arms to steady yourself, but avoid pushing with them.

keep your pelvis stable during a leg-raise exercise, and the hip flexors lift and move your legs.

Problems can occur if your abdominals are too weak to keep your pelvis and lower back stable. If your back arches, this is a sign that you are cheating and potentially causing damage elsewhere, including the joints of the lower back, resulting in increased pain or injury.

It is helpful to strengthen the entire trunk region before engaging in this activity. Placing your hands under your tailbone is a way to help keep the body positioned correctly.

Bent Knee Raise Start

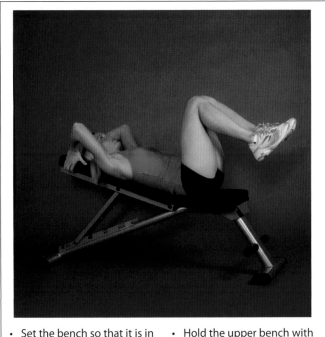

- Set the bench so that it is in a moderate incline position.

- Lie on your back with your hips at the lower end.

- Hold the upper bench with your hands.

- Place your legs together, bend your knees.

Bent Knee Raise Finish

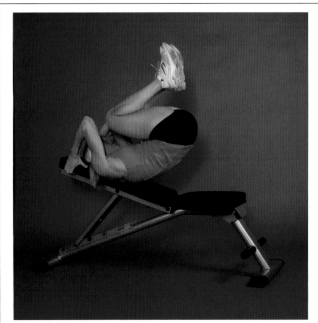

- Lift your feet by using your abdominals.

- Avoid changing the angle of knees once you start raising your feet.

- Follow an arc in your movement.

- Crunch your knees to your chest.

V-UP FAMILY

V-ups are an advanced form of abdominal exercise that require balance and precision to perfect

V-ups, core strength, and Pilates go hand in hand. Pilates is a form of exercise developed by German-born Joseph Pilates. He studied many forms of self-improvement and developed floor exercises, originally for rehabilitation, the prevention of disease, and injury. Today, Pilates is a widely accepted practice that stretches and strengthens your core body muscles,

improving posture and blood circulation.

There are six essential principles central to Pilates: *Centering* your body by focusing on the powerhouse, or the area between your lower ribs and pubic bone. The core, energetically speaking, is the center from which all exercise begins. *Concentration* is bringing full attention to the exercise or movement. *Control*

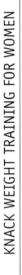

One-Leg Teaser Start

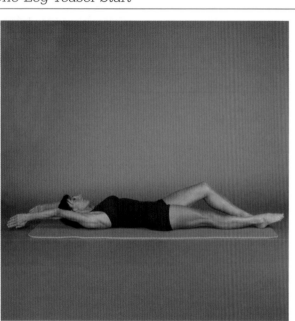

- Lie on your back. Engage your transversus abdominis muscles.

- Extend your arms over your head with legs straight and extended.

- Bend one knee slightly and prepare for movement.

One-Leg Teaser Finish

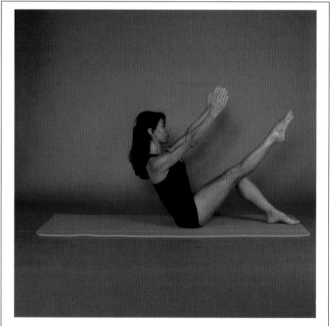

- Keeping your arms straight, lift your upper body, using your abdominals, and balance on your sit bones.

- Reach slowly until your arms are extended in front of you.

- Lift the straight leg until it's even with the bent knee, forming a V shape.

of each movement means no bouncing or swinging. *Precision* and attention to body placement throughout each movement ensure that alignment relative to other body parts is perfected. *Fullness of breath* uses the lungs to pump air fully in and out of the body. *Flow* uses fluidity and grace as they are applied to all exercises and connects all body parts.

Mat Pilates looks similar to traditional abdominal routines. The abdominal exercise called the V-up is referred to as the Teaser and Full Teaser in Pilates. We are going to practice V-ups as if we were Joseph Pilates–trained disciples.

Full Teaser Start

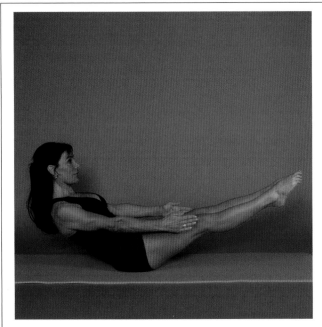

- Lie on your back with both legs extended in front of you.

- Start with your arms by your sides.

- Engage your transversus abdominis muscles. Using your abdominals, lift or scoop your body slowly off the mat.

- Keep your upper body lengthened and your legs reaching away from you.

Full Teaser Finish

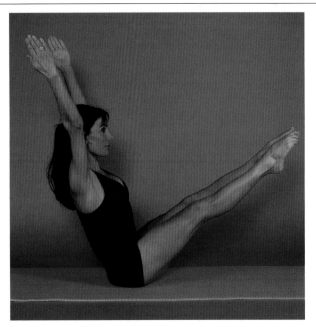

- Continue lifting or scooping your torso and legs to the center position.

- Lift your arms over your head, creating a full V, balancing on your sit bones.

- Hold for a moment; focus on breathing, balance, and body control.

53

OBLIQUES

Side bends will not make your waist smaller or reduce any fat to the area

Strong abdominals equate to a stronger back and a more powerful physique. The obliques, those side muscles that provide abdominal stabilization, body rotation, and side bending, are often a challenging problem for women's fitness goals.

To target the obliques, the best exercise includes rotational movement instead of lateral movement. Rotational exercises develop a smaller waist versus thicker girth. The bicycle crunch and twisting exercises are perfect choices to give you an hourglass figure. Old-fashioned side bends compress the sides of your stomach and work your lower back rather than your obliques. They will make your waist thicker, so avoid them when training.

Bicycle Start

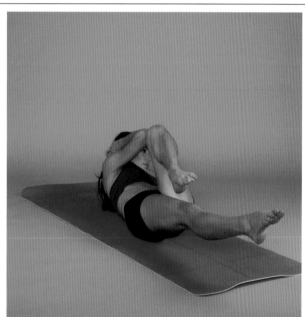

- Lie on your back with neutral spine. Engage your abdominals.

- Place your hands behind your head.

- Bring your left knee up to-ward your right elbow, twisting and lifting your torso.

- Keep your right leg extended in front of you.

- Continue lengthening your head and spine.

Bicycle Finish

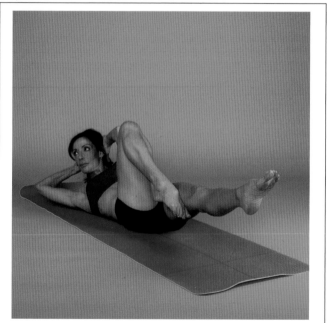

- Bring your right knee up to meet your left elbow, twisting and lifting your torso.

- Your left leg is now extended.

- Continue lengthening your head and spine and engaging your abdominals.

- Repeat this bicycle pedal motion.

54

Any rotational exercise in which you are off your feet will increase the effectiveness of the exercise. When standing, your legs provide strength and stability to the movement. Sitting or lying down forces the effort to be transferred to the oblique and core specifically.

High-frequency training of abdominal muscles, meaning hundreds and hundreds of repetitions daily, is not the solution for getting a smaller waist. To get defined abs, keep up the diet, weights, and cardio training, too.

Russian Twist Start

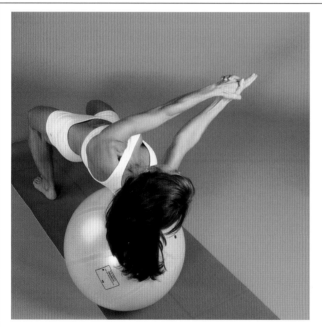

- Start by sitting on a ball.

- Walk your feet forward until head and upper back are supported, hips parallel to shoulders.

- Place hands together,

pointing toward the ceiling.

- Rotate your body to your right side until your left shoulder slightly lifts off the ball.

- Keep hips stationary.

Russian Twist Finish

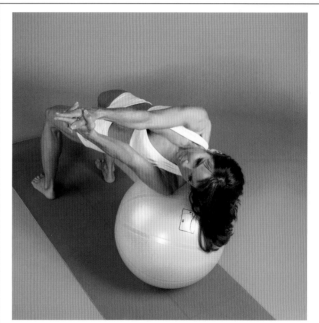

- Without changing the position of your hips and feet, rotate your body to your left side until your right shoulder slightly lifts off the ball.

- Repeat this side-to-side twisting with slow, controlled motion.

CORE CONDITIONING

PLANK

The plank is a measurable assessment of lower abdominal strength and posture that also builds muscle tone

The plank is an isometric exercise and an effective way to tone the abdominals, arms, shoulders, back, and spine. Isometrics are a type of strength training that uses a static position, in that the joint angle and muscle length do not change during contraction. In a plank, the position of the spine does not change.

Isometrics are phenomenal for increasing core stabilization and targeting the transversus abdominus. The critical point to remember during this exercise is to pull your belly button in toward your spine and stay in alignment. Doing so will counter the gravitational force that pulls your body down.

You can perform a modified plank by balancing on your

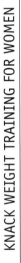

Side Plank Crunch Start

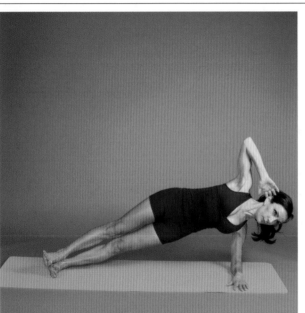

- Lift your body off the floor and balance on one forearm and side of foot.

- Place your other hand gently behind your head, with your elbow to the ceiling, eyes forward.

- Contract your abdominals and relax your shoulders.

- There is no movement. Hold the pose for five to ten seconds.

Side Plank Crunch Finish

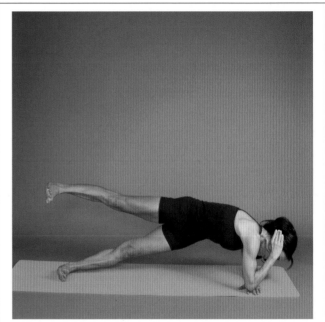

- Lift your top leg into the air as close to hip height as possible while maintaining balance.

- Rotate your torso and bring your elbow to the mat

without moving your lower body. Eyes gaze down.

- Return to start position.

- Repeat on the other side.

elbows and knees, either in a facedown (prone) or side position. This takes moderate coordination and balance to accomplish, making it a great exercise for beginners and intermediates.

Plank variations are abundant, and small changes increase the intensity of the exercise. Lifting one leg off the floor will increase the challenge of the isometric exercise. To transform the plank into a compound movement, pick up a leg and add a crunch action. This position makes the movement dynamic.

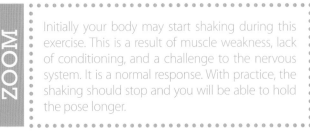
Plank Knee Crunch

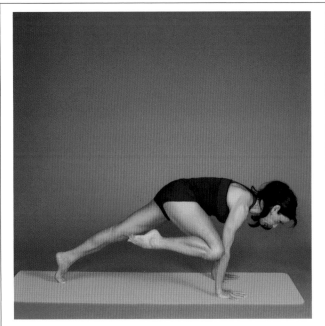

- Lie facedown on the mat, palms on the floor. Push off the floor, arms straight, elbows soft. Rise up to your toes.

- Keep your back lifted and hips even or slightly higher.

- Engage your abdominals.

- Bend knee toward your torso. Tap outside elbow of same-side arm.

- Repeat with other leg and arm.

Plank Cross Knee Crunch

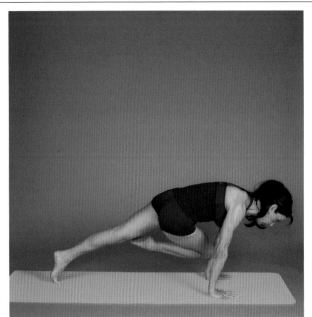

- Repeat plank knee crunch position.

- Bend your knee toward torso. Tap outside of opposite side arm.

- These two variations can be done separately or combined.

- Always extend leg after each elbow tap.

CORE CONDITIONING

WOODCHOPPER AND ROLL

Learn to swing, twist, and extend the torso with greater physical strength

No trees will be cut down or harmed in the course of performing a woodchopper exercise. The name simply refers to a motion by which you propel your body in a movement that mimics that of a lumberjack swinging an axe. Any sport or activity that involves rotational and bending movements with an upright torso requires strength in the midsection. This ex-

ercise will also help prepare your body for more demanding squats and lunges.

The expression *you swing like a girl* originated from women lacking the power and agility to swing forcefully and with conviction. Let's fix that. Woodchoppers can be done using lateral or vertical movement. Use a cable, elastic toner, medi-

Woodchopper Start

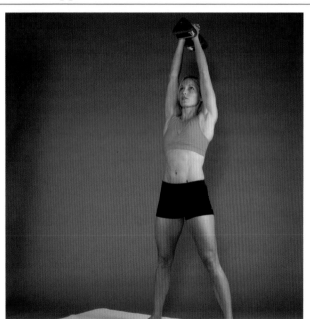

- Assume a wide stance position. Squat to grab the dumbbell. Engage your abdominals.

- Keeping torso straight, bend your knees and swing the dumbbell over your head until your arms are extended and body upright.

- Pause at the top of the movement.

Woodchopper Finish

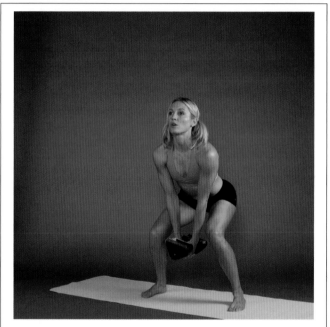

- Lower the dumbbell by bending your knees and sitting back on your heels until the dumbbell reaches the floor between your legs.

- Keep every up-down motion controlled yet explosive.

- Always keep your upper body straight, arms extended, and abdominals engaged.

- Variation: Swing diagonally using a cable or elastic toner.

cine ball, small stability ball, or dumbbell for resistance. You can perform woodchoppers while standing, seated, or kneeling to add variety. Regardless of the variation, it is crucial to keep your arms straight and abs engaged and your lower body stabilized, absorbing the weight transfer as needed. Make each movement explosive yet controlled.

Whereby the woodchopper crunches the midsection, the forward ball roll extends and elongates the abs. This exercise is a functional training staple for the core. The forward roll works the balance muscles of the lower back similarly to the

plank. However, it does so more dynamically.

Proper form is vital to getting the maximum benefit from a forward ball roll. When done correctly, the exercise will increase your level of neuromuscular coordination. Neuromuscular coordination is the harmonious functioning of muscles or muscle groups in the execution of movement. It's the finesse that is visible when someone makes an action look easy even when we know it's not!

Forward Ball Roll Start

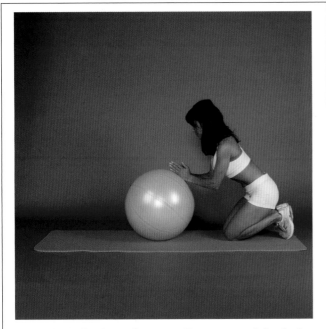

- Place the ball in front of you and kneel behind it; tuck toes under feet.

- Place your palms together on top of the ball, close to the body. Your elbows should be bent 90 degrees.

- Engage your abdominals while keeping your upper body straight. Keep head in line with spine.

Forward Ball Roll Finish

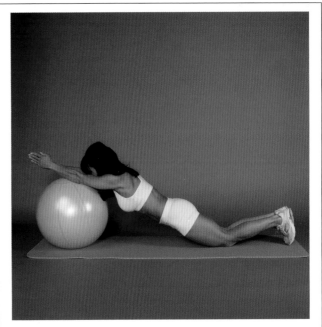

- Roll the ball forward by extending your arms. Maintain proper spine alignment.

- Use your abs to pull the ball back to start position.

- Focus on using your abs, not your arms, to roll out and back.

- Readjust your hands when in kneeling position, as they tend to shift.

WIDE PUSH-UP

Doing one push-up *perfectly* is better than doing ten push-ups with weakness and sloppy form

The wide push-up is the closest thing there is to a perfect resistance exercise. Push-ups are versatile and can be performed anywhere, anytime. They work muscles in the entire body, including the shoulders, arms, back, core, hips, and legs. The push-up is a convenient exercise to increase your bone density.

Push-ups are a challenging, advanced fitness exercise and can be modified for beginners. Any wall, chair, countertop, or floor can be a training tool. You don't need special clothes or a lot of time to bust out a few repetitions!

During a floor push-up, you lift about half your body weight, so it's impressively powerful training when done correctly. To do a push-up perfectly takes core strength and preexisting

Wide Push-up Start

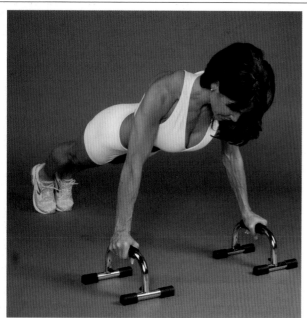

- Push-up handles reduce wrist stress. Handles allow the chest to drop deeper for more challenge.

- Wide arm position start: Hips and waist are straight. Engage your abdominals.

- Push through the heels, lengthen your spine and neck.

- Use your arms, back, and chest as primary muscle movers.

Wide Push-up Finish

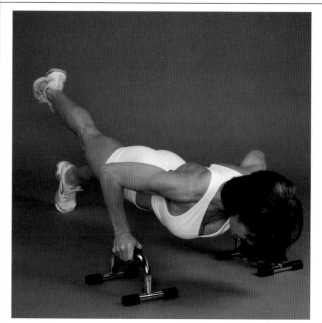

- Lower your upper body to the floor.

- Pause at the bottom. Your chest will not touch the floor.

- Lift one leg off floor to progress.

- For an easier variation, place your hands on a wall or countertop.

fitness. Building up to a push-up is easy if you practice a plank pose daily. The plank exercise increases the stabilizer-muscle strength needed to perform a push-up without cheating. Be sure to keep your body alignment straight, hips lifted, and your arms and elbows in the plane of movement that maintains correct form.

If a regular push-up is too difficult, start with wall push-ups, then progress to using a countertop or modified floor push-up by resting on your knees. More advanced options include a floor push-up with one leg raised.

GREEN ● LIGHT

Aim for ten perfect push-ups. Then a goal should be to *do as many as your age every day* for good measure. Push-ups are recommended as *part* of your daily routine. However, they will not work your pull muscles, nor will they build cardiovascular fitness needed for heart health and extra calorie burning. So, consider them a cross-training and stability-building exercise. They're fantastic!

Incline Push-up Start

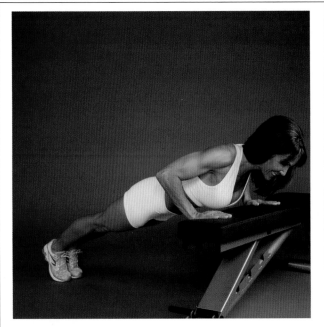

- Wide arm position start on the side of bench.

- Hips and waist are straight. Engage your abdominals.

- With toes on the floor, push body up with arms extended.

- Lower your body back to the bench and immediately push the body up as fast as possible.

Incline Push-up Clap

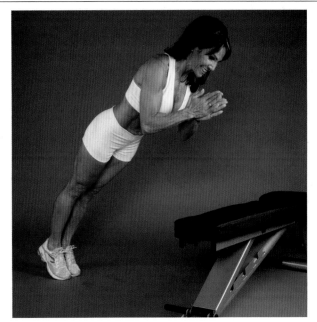

- Keep hips and waist straight.

- As the hands leave the bench, rapidly clap them together and then place them back to original posi-

tion, catching your body before it falls.

- For even more challenge, increase the number of claps between push-ups.

STABILITY PUSH-UP

Doing a push-up on a stability ball will work more muscles than a floor push-up

Take your push-up fitness to another level with a stability ball. No longer will all your points of contact be on a solid surface. Either your hands or your feet will be exposed to an unstable environment, forcing more of your muscle fibers to activate, including your core.

With a stability ball you will need to balance, focus your

mind, maintain stability, and move up and down without deviating from proper form. Stability balls allow for a greater range of motion and different angles to be added to the exercise. The round ball allows you to hold your hands lower than you would on the floor or a wall and permits alignment modifications.

Stability Push-up Start

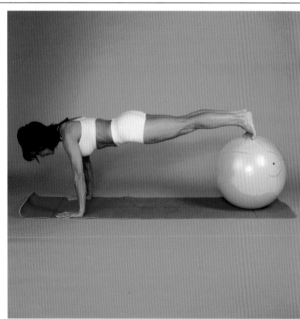

- Position your belly or shins on the ball and hands on the floor.

- Walk your hands forward until your toes are on top of the ball.

- Maintain neutral body position.

- Support your upper body with extended arms, shoulder-width apart in plank position.

Stability Push-up Finish

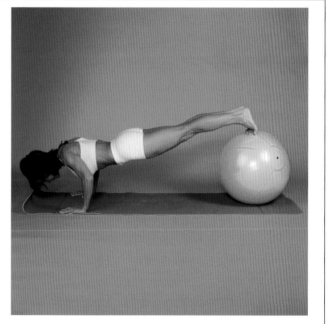

- Lower your upper body to the floor by bending your elbows.

- Keep hips and waist straight and continue to engage your core.

- Chest does not touch the floor.

Tackle the stability ball after you have mastered the ability to do ten to twenty traditional push-ups. Be prepared to feel humbled at first, and have a towel on hand, as you are sure to perspire! The nervous system will be in overdrive as you activate your muscles in a wobbly situation.

Don't overdo the first couple attempts, and make sure that you have a spotter or are working on a soft surface, in case you roll off.

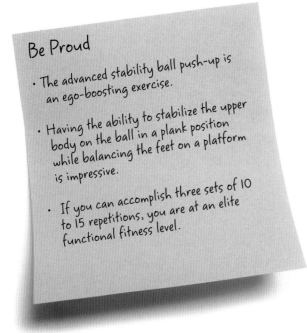

Be Proud

• The advanced stability ball push-up is an ego-boosting exercise.

• Having the ability to stabilize the upper body on the ball in a plank position while balancing the feet on a platform is impressive.

• If you can accomplish three sets of 10 to 15 repetitions, you are at an elite functional fitness level.

MAKE IT EASY

The secret to becoming really proficient with a stability ball is developing your fundamental skills little by little. Practice sitting on a ball. Lift one foot off the floor and keep the ball from moving. Become comfortable lying on the ball from all angles. You might also want to use a stability ball while sitting at your desk for part of the day.

Advanced Stability Push-up

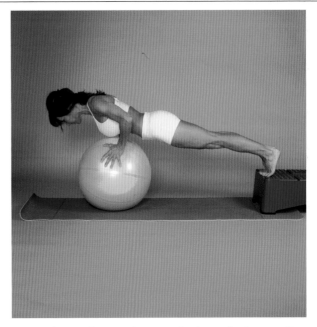

• Lay with your chest on the stability ball. Place hands on the ball at the sides of your chest. Keep legs straight and feet on a step or bench.

• Push your body up until your arms are straight. Do not lock your elbows.

• Lower down until elbows are at 90 degrees or just before your chest touches the ball.

CHEST PRESS

The dumbbell chest press is a highly effective movement for toning and shaping the upper body

The chest press is a classic exercise. Nicely developed chest muscles on a woman help shape the cleavage and add a firm foundation for the breasts. To train the chest a stability ball, bench, and dumbbells can be incorporated.

The muscles of the chest are the pectoralis major and, below it, the pectoralis minor. The muscles are large and fan shaped,

running across the upper portion of the rib cage and toward the shoulder. A chest-press exercise recruits from secondary muscles, including the shoulders, triceps (back of arms), and trapezius (traps). The traps are the diamond-shaped muscles at the base of the neck that run down the middle of the back. These muscles are important because many women com-

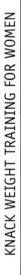

Chest Press Start

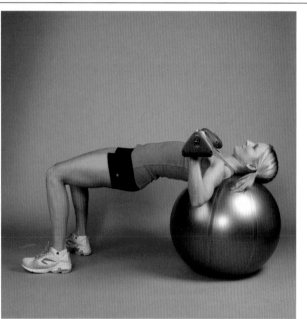

- Sit upright on the ball, feet flat on the floor. Walk forward, allowing the ball to roll underneath your body.

- Upper back on the ball, hips parallel to floor, retract your

shoulders and engage your core.

- Hold dumbbells with palms forward, next to the chest, elbows out to sides.

Chest Press Finish

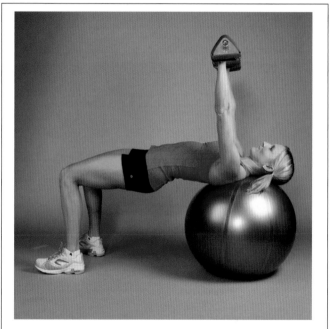

- Keep the body stable, chest high, shoulders retracted.

- Extend and press arms toward the ceiling.

- Hands are shoulder-width apart. Do not lock elbows.

- Lower the dumbbells by bending your elbows.

plain of tension in this area, often caused by overuse, lack of mobility, and poor posture.

Dumbbells provide a means to improve symmetry and balance in both arms during the lift portion of the chest press. Move both arms evenly, using the same amount of weight to avoid one arm being stronger or more dominant than the other.

Honor your form when practicing this exercise by learning to retract your shoulders properly. The shoulders and traps should be a secondary helper, not the main form of power.

Incline Chest Press

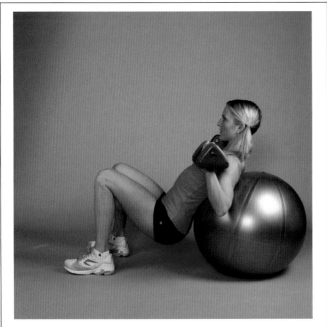

- Sit upright, feet flat on floor. Walk forward, allowing ball to roll underneath your body.

- Mid to upper back on the ball, hips dropped to the floor, retract your shoulders and engage your core.

- Dumbbells in hands next to your chest, keep elbows to your sides. Press arms toward the ceiling. Lower.

Decline Chest Press

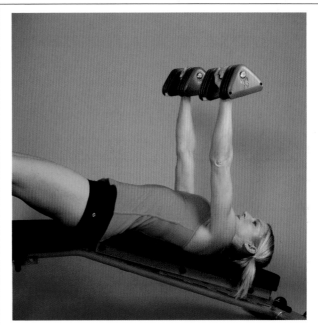

- This exercise cannot be performed on a ball.

- Grab weights while sitting up, hold them against your chest, and ease into a decline position.

- Press arms toward ceiling and lower dumbbells by bending elbows.

- After each set, roll up, holding weights against your body, or rotate upper body to ease dumbbells to floor.

THE FLY

Strengthening the chest muscles can lift the breasts, firming and enhancing the bustline

It is aesthetically pleasing to have nice chest muscles. A strong chest is practical, too. The chest muscles improve posture.

Because we tend to spend so many hours on our computers, with our hands forward, shoulders slouched, and neck looking out over papers, the chest muscles shorten and become tighter. Over time this decreases mobility and creates imbalances within the body. It negatively affects our backs, which weakens as a result.

A well-developed chest needs exercises to strengthen the upper and lower pectoral muscles. The flat, incline, and decline chest press form a perfect combination of training elements for improvement. The fly exercise offers more advancement.

Fly Start

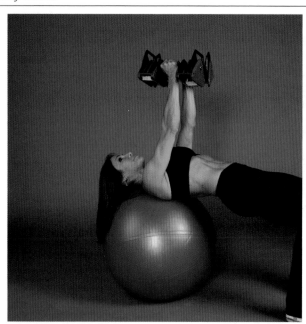

- Sit upright on a ball, feet flat on the floor. Walk forward, allowing the ball to roll underneath your body.

- Keeping your upper back on the ball and hips parallel to floor, retract shoulders and engage your core.

- Raise the dumbbells above your chest with palms facing each other.

- Elbows are slightly bent.

Fly Finish

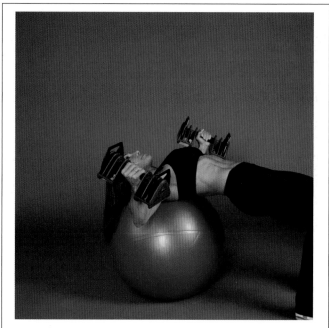

- Keep your elbows only slightly bent. Lower the dumbbells in an arching motion.

- Keep your arms in a horizontal plane at your nipple-line.

- Lower your upper arms to parallel or slightly past parallel to floor.

- Return by maintaining a slight bend in your arms throughout the movement.

The dumbbell fly does not involve the triceps, as does the compound chest-press exercise. It will recruit the biceps, as well as the shoulders. Because your arm is in an extended position during a fly, you won't be able to lift as much weight compared to a chest press.

Even though the fly is an everyday movement similar to giving a large friend a big hug, the exercise must be taught, as there are nuances to correct form. Watch for warning signs of poor form, like recruiting from the trapezius and hunching the shoulders.

MAKE IT EASY

Practice the motion of the fly in front of a mirror. With shoulders retracted, abdominals engaged, and neck long, mimic the arm position of a ballet dancer whose fingers of both hands are almost touching to form an oval at chest level. Open your arms wide without pinching the shoulder blades, keeping your elbows parallel to the floor at chest level.

Incline Fly

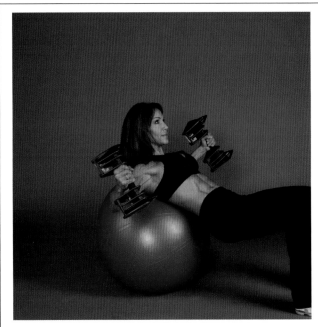

- Sit upright on the ball, feet flat on the floor. Walk forward, allowing the ball to roll underneath your body.

- Mid to upper back on the ball, hips dropped to floor, retract your shoulders and engage your core.

- Use same arm motion as flat fly.

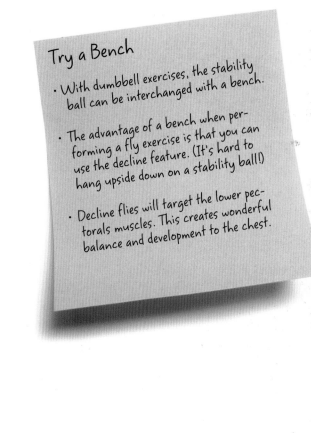

Try a Bench

- With dumbbell exercises, the stability ball can be interchanged with a bench.

- The advantage of a bench when performing a fly exercise is that you can use the decline feature. (It's hard to hang upside down on a stability ball!)

- Decline flies will target the lower pectorals muscles. This creates wonderful balance and development to the chest.

CROSSOVERS

Teeing off in golf and hitting a forehand in tennis use crossover movements

Weight lifters regard the cable crossover exercise as the finishing school for the chest. It is a single-joint movement that isolates your pectoralis muscle (pecs). If you are lean, you may notice striations in your chest, especially when you hold your hands back over your head. The cable crossover exercise develops those striations.

You can use an elastic toner for this exercise. It provides a smooth, enjoyable muscular action. It is best to do the cable crossover at the end of your chest workout, once the main muscle group that you have isolated is fatigued. This is one of those exercises where you will feel the burn. Having a cable or elastic toner provides just the progressive resistance to keep

Cable Crossover Start

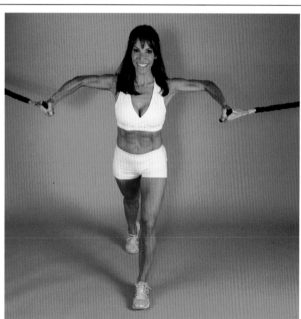

- Anchor one toner overhead or two equal toners at opposite side points.

- Grab the handles, palms facing each other.

- In neutral position, step ahead of the anchor points, angling your upper body forward 30 degrees.

- With arms fixed in a slightly bent position at chest level, internally rotate shoulders, keeping elbows wide.

Cable Crossover Finish

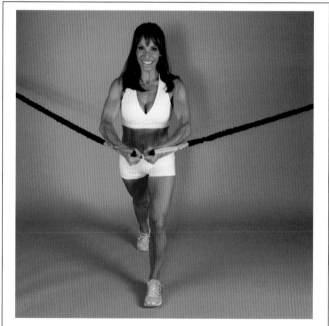

- Pull (don't press) toners together in a hugging motion. Aim for a spot away from but level with your belly button, palms facing each other.

- Keep shoulders retracted, elbows fixed, wrists straight.

- Pull equally on both sides, working your chest muscles.

- To target your pecs, anchor the toners low.

the muscles working throughout the entire movement.

The finish position of the crossover resembles a hand clap in front of your body, or a full scissor effect where the arms cross over each other. If you employ the scissor-arm technique, make sure you alternate by crossing the right arm over the left on one rep, and the left arm over the right on the next rep. The extra range of motion provides maximum muscle activation. When getting started, it may be easier to simply meet the hands in the middle.

Reverse Low Crossover Start

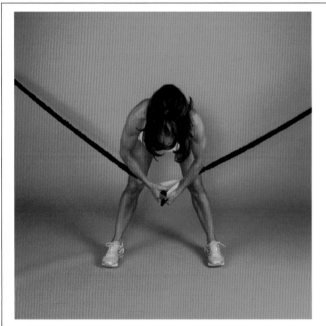

- This is a rear-deltoid (shoulder) exercise where the upper chest plays an antagonist role.

- Use a wide stance and bend forward with neutral body position. Slightly bend your elbows.

- Start with hands together in front of your body. Left hand holds the right cable, right hand holds the left cable.

Reverse Low Crossover Finish

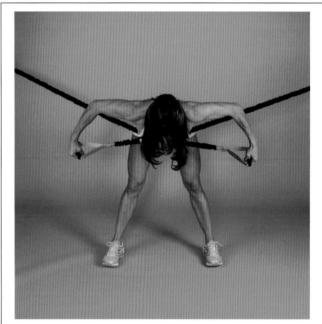

- Keep your back straight and body bent over, with torso parallel to the floor.

- Pull back, extending arms straight out to either side and crossing cables in front of your body. Turn wrists slightly, thumbs down.

- Stretch as far as possible. Return arms in controlled hugging motion focusing on the chest.

PULL-OVER AND CABLE PULL

Women benefit from well-rounded chest exercises that improve posture and balance the body

The pull-over and cable pull utilize dumbbells and a cable or elastic toner for resistance. These exercises add variety and target the chest in yet another way. They also incorporate some of the back muscles, helping keep both sides of your body balanced.

The pull-over targets the serratus anterior muscle and pec-

torals. The serratus anterior muscle originates on the surface of the upper ribs, as well as the side of the chest, and inserts along the length of the shoulder blade. If you place the palms of your hands up and near your armpits, and fan your fingers toward your breasts, you are on top of the serratus anterior muscles.

Pull-over Start

Pull-over Finish

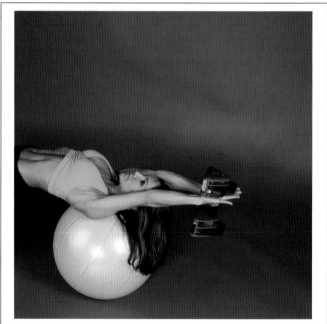

- Sit upright, feet flat on the floor. Walk forward, allowing the ball to roll underneath your body.

- Upper back on the ball, hips parallel to the floor, retract your shoulders and engage your core.

- Hold the top of the dumbbell with palms.

- Raise the dumbbell above your chest, with straight arms.

- Keeping arms straight, lower the dumbbell slowly in an arc behind your head.

- Connect your rib cage, while feeling the stretch.

- Lower the dumbbell as much as possible.

- Raise back to start position without using your hips to help.

The pull-over is known for expanding the rib cage, which helps create a V-shaped upper body. It's a critical muscle for self-defense. Often called the boxer's muscle, it helps you throw a punch. A weakness in the serratus anterior muscles can also create back issues. When performing the pull-over, it's imperative to engage your abdominals and connect the rib cage. You'll know your rib cage is not connected if your ribs poke out instead of staying flat against your torso.

The cable pull exercise is another example of an exercise that targets the serratus muscles and hits the abs and latissimus dorsi (lats). The lats are the largest muscle in the upper body, are triangular in shape, and extend from your shoulders down either side of the small of your back. From an application standpoint, we use our lats a lot for lifting and pulling. It is easy to only feel this exercise in that muscle location. Focus on the serratus muscles (visualize where they are during the exercise), as this should help isolate them. Maintain strict form.

Cable Pull Start

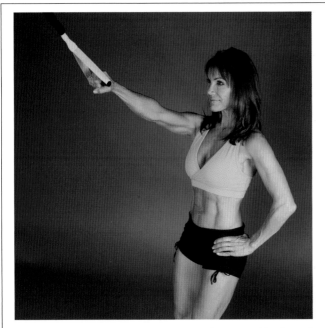

- Also called One-Arm Press Down.

- Anchor the toner over your head. Stand facing the anchor and grab the handle, palm facing down.

- Stand in neutral body position.

- Core engagement here is key to prevent your body from swaying or rocking.

Cable Pull Finish

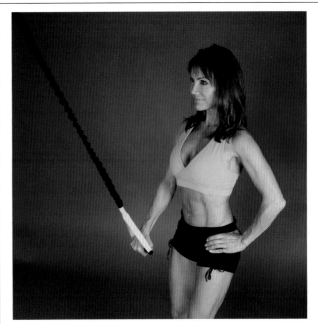

- From standing position, pull toner down toward your leg by using your back (lats) and chest (serratus) muscles.

- Release the cable slowly,

focusing attention on your serratus muscle.

- Variations: Use kneeling position. Do both arms at the same time.

EXTENSION AND HYPEREXTENSION

The term *posterior chain* describes the glutes, hamstrings, and lower back as a functional unit

According to the American Academy of Orthopedic Surgeons, four out of five adults experience or will experience lower-back pain at some point in their lives. Common general reasons include a lack of core strength, poor flexibility, and poor posture. Obesity can also cause or exacerbate back problems. Sitting in a chair or car for a large portion of the day tightens the hamstrings and hip flexors (iliopsoas muscle) and fatigues the muscles that support the spine.

Training your posterior chain may improve the situation. The erector spinae are the back muscles on either side of the spine. They are arranged in three vertical columns and are the chief extensors of the spinal column. Deeper yet are

Back Extension Start

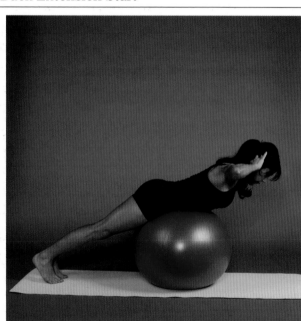

- Start on your knees, ball in front. Plant feet on the mat.

- Place your stomach on the ball and straighten legs with majority of your weight on ball.

- Align your upper and lower body. Place hands behind ears, elbows out to your sides.

- Hands across your chest or behind your back are easier options.

Back Extension Finish

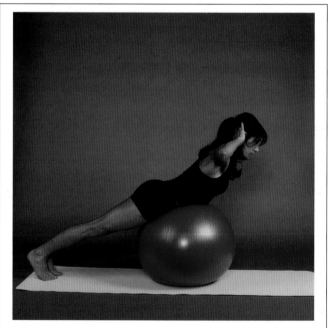

- Squeeze your buttocks and raise your upper body without arching your back and compressing discs.

- Engage your abdominals.

- Pause at the top of the movement, then lower your body forward over the ball.

muscles that help rotate the body, flex and extend the trunk, and stabilize the vertebra.

We can improve the development of all these muscles and make them stronger using a stability ball. Hyperextensions and reverse hyperextensions work the buttocks and hamstrings, so the benefit to the bottom half of the body is twofold. Strength in this region will assist in virtually every lower-body, back-specific exercise and core movement.

BACK

Reverse Hyperextension Start

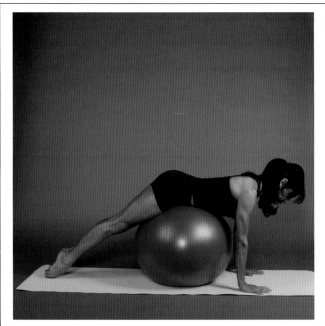

- Lie with your belly on the ball with palms flat on the mat. Legs are straight, resting on top of your toes.

- Retract shoulders, engage core, and maintain neutral spine.

Reverse Hyperextension Finish

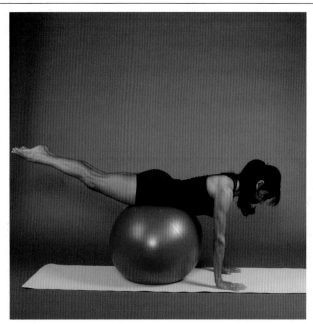

- Keeping legs together and straight, lift them up until level or slightly higher than your hips.

- Pause and lower legs back down, lightly touching toes to the floor.

- Do not swing legs up or drop them down.

- Keep abdominals engaged and maintain neutral spine.

73

SWIMMING AND SUPERMAN

Keep your back in a neutral position and avoid any rotation throughout the movement

The erector spinae is a bundle of muscles running down the sides of the vertebral column on your back. These muscles can become tight from inactivity, poor posture, and lack of stretching. They may feel literally fused together. This is not the case, but this feeling indicates that exercise and flexibility are needed to keep your body's fascia healthy and pliable.

Fascia is the soft-tissue component of the connective-tissue system in the body. It is like a web around the muscles, bones, nerves, and blood vessels. The fascia is responsible for maintaining the structural integrity of the body, providing support and protection and acting as a shock absorber.

Deep fascia can contract and is part of the flight-or-fight

Swimming Start

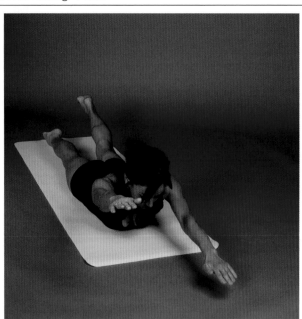

Swimming Finish

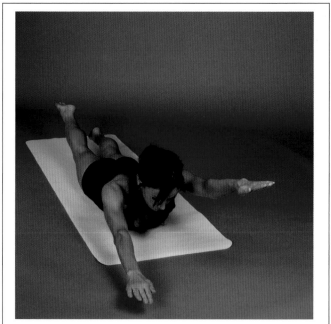

- Lie on your belly with legs straight and together.

- Retract your shoulders and stretch your arms straight overhead.

- Engage your abdominals, lengthen your spine.

- Lift right arm and left leg off the mat, keeping your face down.

- Do not crease your neck. Keep tailbone tucked.

- Maintain body position.

- Switch and lift right leg and left arm.

- Keep alternating, pumping up and down in small pulses.

response. Bolstered with tensioned fascia, people are able to perform extraordinary feats of strength and speed under emergency conditions. How fascia contracts is still not well understood. The important point is that fascia is part of the powerful human process that we should keep in shape.

Your erector spinea and the surrounding fascia will maintain healthy function by combining specific exercises, such as swimming and superman routines, along with flexibility and/or deep tissue massage therapy.

YELLOW ●LIGHT

Generally speaking, large-muscle, multi-joint exercises should be trained first during a workout session, followed by single-muscle isolation exercises. This prevents early fatigue. Since your back muscles are used in many exercises as a stabilizer, doing low-back-specific hyperextensions at the end of a workout is the safer choice.

Superman

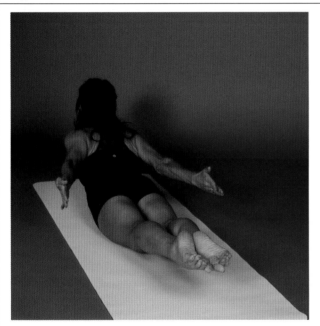

- Lie on your belly, arms extended back, and rotate your palms up.

- Simultaneously lift your head, upper back, arms, and legs off the mat.

- Keep legs together and extended. Retract shoulders and engage abdominals.

- Hold pose for five seconds. Slowly lower, resting body on the mat.

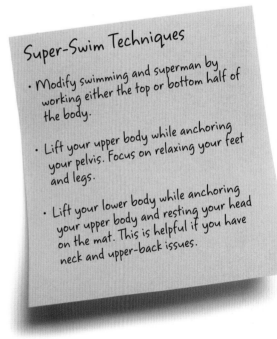

Super-Swim Techniques

- Modify swimming and superman by working either the top or bottom half of the body.

- Lift your upper body while anchoring your pelvis. Focus on relaxing your feet and legs.

- Lift your lower body while anchoring your upper body and resting your head on the mat. This is helpful if you have neck and upper-back issues.

LAT PULL-DOWN

Pull-down exercises are hard to duplicate at home without an elastic toner

The pull-down exercise is meant to develop the latissimus dorsi (lats), the largest muscle in the back. If you like the broad shoulder, small waist physique, this is the movement for you. It is a compound exercise, which means it works more than one muscle at the same time. The pull-down trains a host of back muscles, including the rhomboids, which are responsi-

ble for retracting the shoulder blades, the erector spinae, the low-back muscles, and the muscles of the arms and shoulders.

In a gym setting, the lat pull-down machine offers options to tweak this exercise. You can choose a different handle and grip position and adjust the weight systematically. A pad-

Lat Pull-Down Start

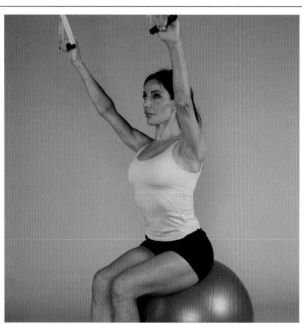

- Anchor the toner overhead. Facing the anchor, grab the handles, palms forward, and hold arms overhead.

- Sit on the ball with neutral body position. Retract your shoulders, engage your abdominals.

- Toner should have some tension to start.

Lat Pull-Down Finish

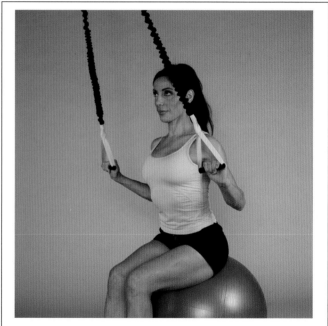

- Keeping neutral spine, pull equally on both handles by bending your elbows.

- Keep your hands, lower arms, and toner in alignment.

- Lower your hands to chest level, elbows out to the sides.

- Avoid overarching your back or moving your arms out of the vertical plane.

76

ded bar to tuck your legs under keeps your lower body anchored.

At home you are limited to elastic toners, because you can't duplicate a lat pull-down with dumbbells. Whether at the gym using a cable machine or at home using an elastic toner, the action of the movement is the same.

Sitting on a stability ball will increase the difficulty of the exercise. Anchor an elastic toner to the top of a door and sit on the ball facing it. Keep your feet flat on the floor and position your hands so that your palms are facing away from you, knuckles up. The move should initiate from your lats by retracting your shoulder blades (putting them in your back pocket) and lowering your elbows toward the floor. Maintain an invisible line from your hands to your elbows to the floor and stay within that plane of motion. If you were to use a wide bar, you would end the motion at the center of your chest, above the breasts.

It is perfectly acceptable to arch the back slightly during this exercise, so long as you connect the rib cage, engage the abdominals, and lengthen the spine.

One-Arm Lat Pull-Down Start

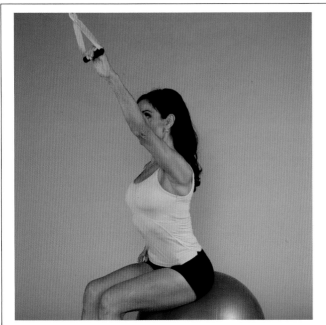

- Use same body position and motion as lat pull-down.

- Take advantage of the increased stretch at the top of the movement. Stretch from your back; avoid extending your shoulder joint and pinching your neck.

- As you stretch, do not let shoulder pull out of its socket; stretch from your back.

One-Arm Lat Pull-Down Finish

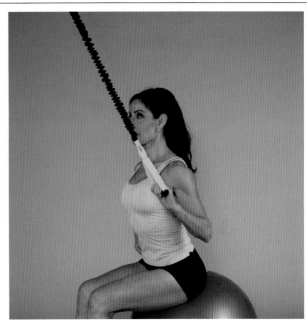

- Maintain forearm alignment with toner. Pull your elbow straight down.

- Always pause for a second at top and bottom so momentum is eliminated.

- Unilateral pull-down isolates one lat at a time.

77

TWO-ARM ROW

Rowing as a sport is a smooth, rhythmic, non-impact motion that offers superior conditioning

Considered one of the best muscle builders for the back and shoulders, the bent-over row is very popular. As with most strength-training exercises for the torso, it improves posture and upper-body strength. Body symmetry requires exercises to be performed on various angles of a muscle group. The bent-over dumbbell row targets the back side of the deltoid,

helping people with shoulder slouch problems and restoring a flattering shape to the muscles.

The bent-over dumbbell row is an approachable exercise for individuals who suffer discomfort while doing specific lower- and upper-back exercises. When you get to a stage where you have increased the dumbbell weight to the point

Bent-over Row Start

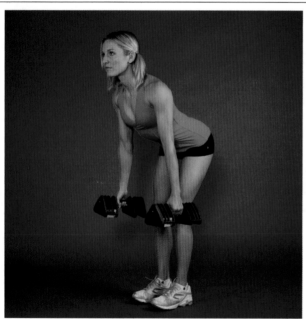

- Hold dumbbells with palms facing each other. Feet shoulder-width apart, knees slightly bent.

- Bend forward from the hips, to a 45-degree angle. Keep your back straight and en-gage your core, retracting your shoulders.

- Let arms hang straight down, with a slight bend in the elbows.

Bent-over Row Finish

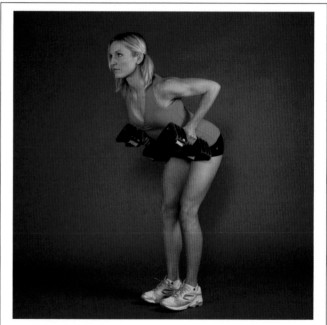

- Lift both dumbbells until level with your back, el-bows toward the ceiling.

- Slowly lower down to the starting point.

- Keep legs and body still throughout the move-ment and keep shoulders retracted.

- Variations: Move one arm at a time. Face palms back.

where your grip falters, consider purchasing hand grips. You can find them on the Internet or at sports stores. Hand grips help reduce forearm pump and strain.

Seated cable rows (at the gym) or elastic-toner seated rows target similar muscles as the bent-over row, also emphasizing the trapezius. Do not be frightened to train the traps. Just remember to do so in correct body alignment, retracting the shoulders so that you are not initiating the movement from your upper neck. The benefit of retraction exercises is that they eliminate rounded shoulders that tend to be pulled forward.

··········· GREEN ● LIGHT ··············

Try a bent-over dumbbell-alternating row. Assume the same position as the two-arm row. Hold dumbbells with a "thumbs in and elbows out" or "palms facing in" grip. Row one dumbbell up to the full range of motion. As you lower it, row the other dumbbell up. Continue with this up-down action so that the dumbbells are always moving in a simultaneous motion.

Seated Row Start

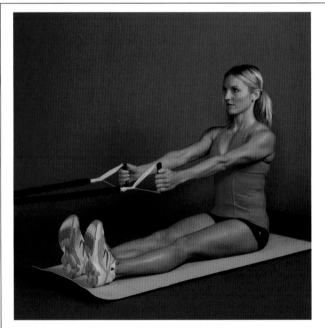

Seated Row Finish

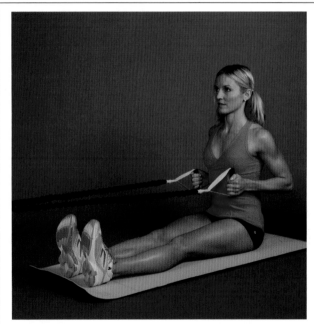

- Anchor toner at chest level. Sit on mat facing the anchor; grab the handles with your palms facing each other.

- Slide hips back; keep knees straight but not locked.

- Maintain neutral body position. Retract your shoulders.

- Start with tension on toner.

- Pull elbows back with equal pressure on both. Keep shoulders retracted and back neutral.

- Return until arms are extended, shoulders stretched forward, and lower back

flexed slightly forward.

- Pause before beginning next rep; do not bounce.

- Variation: Palms down and elbows out to sides.

BOW AND ARROW

When strengthening specific muscles, include right and left sides, which provides balance and symmetry

The bow-and-arrow exercise mimics the movement of an archer. It is an upper-body exercise that relies on lower-body balance to keep you steady. You will work the upper-back and shoulder muscles to draw the elastic toner and control it, then the arm muscles to extend the elastic toner, while rotating the torso and stabilizing the spine.

Standing rotational movements offer greater benefit to your body than their seated counterparts. The simultaneous movement of pulling with opposite arms and altering foot placement creates a muscle-group sequencing challenge that duplicates the complex muscle demands of everyday life. During a standing rotational movement, your lower back

Bow and Arrow: Right Start

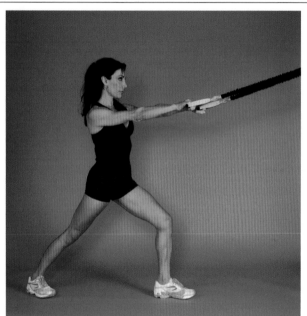

- Anchor the toner overhead. Stand facing the anchor. Grab handles with palms down.

- Lunge right leg back. Center weight in neutral body position. Engage abdominals and retract shoulders.

- Extend the arms and align them with the toner.

- Start with tension on the elastic.

Bow and Arrow: Right Finish

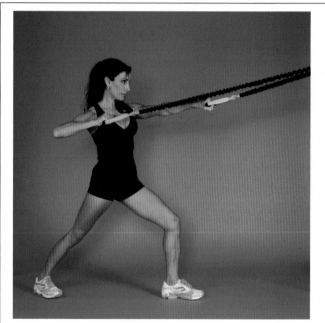

- Pull right hand to chest by bringing elbow straight back. Maintain alignment of right lower arm and the toner.

- Rotate your torso slightly during contraction. Keep shoulders retracted.

- Your back is the primary mover.

is less vulnerable because you aren't putting undo pressure on the intervertebral discs of the lumbar spine.

Archery as a sport demands focus and mental preparation, along with physical strength. The same principle can apply to the elastic toner exercise. Anchor the toner with enough tension so that you feel the progressive loading gains. Focus your mind on your breathing, inhaling through your nose and exhaling through your mouth. Feel your body move gracefully and with precision throughout each repetition. Always keep your eye on the target.

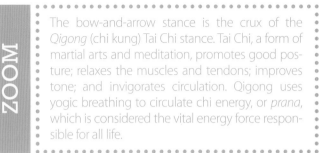

The bow-and-arrow stance is the crux of the *Qigong* (chi kung) Tai Chi stance. Tai Chi, a form of martial arts and meditation, promotes good posture; relaxes the muscles and tendons; improves tone; and invigorates circulation. Qigong uses yogic breathing to circulate chi energy, or *prana*, which is considered the vital energy force responsible for all life.

Bow and Arrow: Left Start

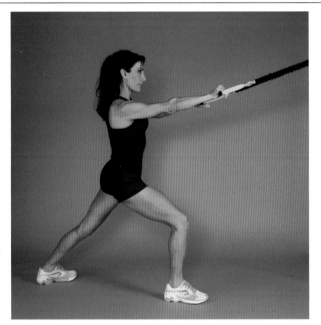

- Keep the anchor overhead and grip with palms down.

- Lunge left leg back. Center your weight in neutral body position. Engage abdominals and retract shoulders.

- Extend your arms and align them with the toner.

- Start with tension on the elastic.

Bow and Arrow: Left Finish

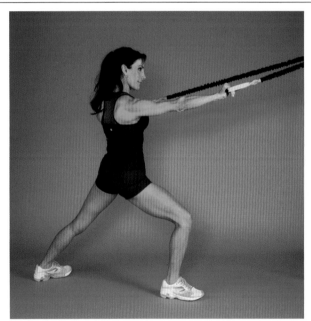

- Follow the same action as on the right side.

- Maximize range of motion by bringing your elbow back as far as possible and releasing so that the back is stretched.

- Maintain body alignment throughout.

GOOD MORNING

This exercise is thusly named because it resembles the movement of formally bowing to greet someone

The good morning exercise strengthens the lower back, glutes, and hamstrings. When properly applied, it reduces injury. The good morning exercise is a stiff-legged, straight-back exercise and tends to scare people away. It carries claims of being a potential cause of lower-back injuries, not an exercise that is beneficial for avoiding them. If you feel intimidated, try a bent-leg, straight-back version.

With both movements it is vital to keep your back straight when bending over and to never twist the spine. A technique to help this lowering move is to keep your chin lifted and eyes focused ahead. Like skiing, the body follows the head. Look where you're going.

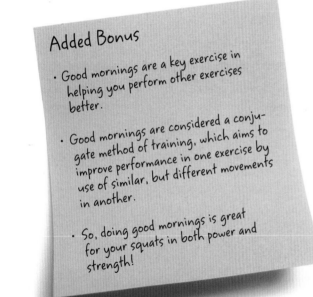

Added Bonus

• Good mornings are a key exercise in helping you perform other exercises better.

• Good mornings are considered a conjugate method of training, which aims to improve performance in one exercise by use of similar, but different movements in another.

• So, doing good mornings is great for your squats in both power and strength!

Good Morning: Position 1

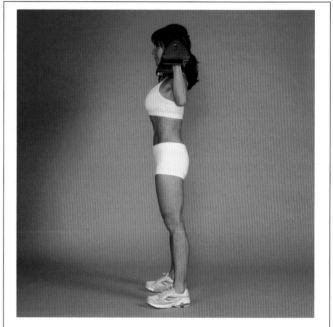

• Stand in neutral body position, feet shoulder-width apart.

• Hold dumbbells with palms forward so they rest evenly on your shoulders.

• Focus eyes forward.

The hips should be the hinge point of the good morning. If you have tight hamstrings, a full range of motion during the exercise may not be achieved. Ideally you should bend forward until your upper body is parallel to the floor. Over-achievers will seek this end position by bending or rounding their upper back to accommodate. This is a bad idea and poor form. Neutral body position doubly applies to the good morning exercise. The low back will retain its natural curve—no less, no more.

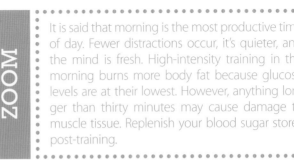
BACK

Good Morning: Position 2

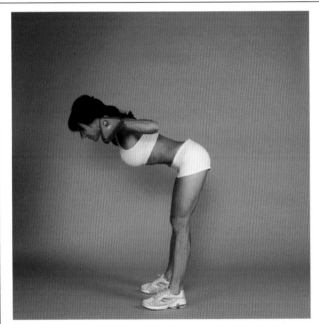

- Without moving dumbbells, gradually bend forward using your hips to lower chest to 45 degrees.

- Keep legs straight, but not locked. Keep weight toward your heels.

- Continue to engage your abdominals.

- Keep your head neutral or look up.

Good Morning: Position 3

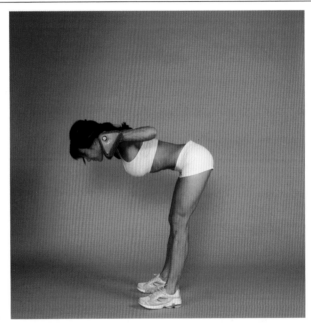

- Continue lowering your chest until your upper body is parallel to the floor.

- Hold for a moment and return.

- If your back rounds when you bend, you may have tight hamstrings and hips. Lower only as far as you can while keeping your back straight with neutral spine.

BICEPS CURL, HAMMER CURL

Curls, a toning exercise, isolate and strengthen the muscles in the upper arms

If you are trying to lose weight, a compound exercise is the best option for burning more calories. Exercises that use multiple large muscle groups at the same time equate to a higher metabolism, helping you reduce fat, tone up, and get leaner. Cardiovascular or aerobic training qualifies as a multi-joint exercise that burns calories effectively, too.

However, isolation exercises have a definitive purpose in a well-balanced, full-body weight-training program. Working one muscle group in an isolated manner helps build specific strength and may be necessary to support more complicated compound exercises. It is often the details that help shape and define us!

Biceps Curl Start

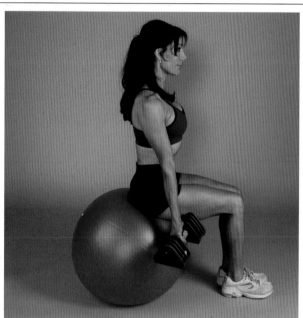

- Sit on the stability ball with your feet flat on the floor and legs together.

- Maintain neutral spine and keep abdominals engaged and shoulders retracted.

- Start with dumbbells by your sides. Palms up, elbows tucked tight to your body.

- Modification: Feet apart offers more stability.

Biceps Curl Finish

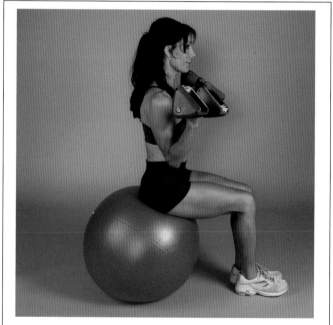

- Keeping elbows tucked to the sides of your body, curl dumbbells up to the shoulders by contracting the biceps.

- Lower the dumbbells slowly back to the start position.

- Flex during eccentric motion (lowering) to recruit more muscle fibers.

The biceps curl is an example of an isolation exercise because it isolates the muscles in your upper arms. Improving the strength of your grip, forearm, and biceps assists when training other body parts, including the back and shoulders. Strong arms come in handy when household projects need some elbow grease!

Hammer curls refer to the position of the hands during the movement. The palms face inward, similar to the shape of a hammer, and stay that way throughout the exercise.

BICEPS

Hammer Curl Mid Position

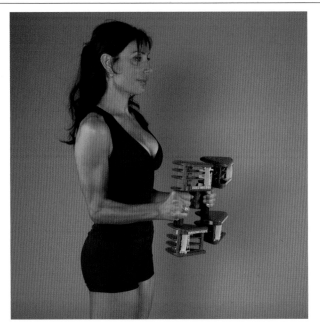

- Stand with legs and feet together in neutral body position. Engage abdominals and retract your shoulders.

- Keep elbows tucked to the sides of your body and your

palms facing each other (hammer position).

- Start with dumbbells hanging by your sides. Lift to mid position by contracting biceps.

Hammer Curl Finish

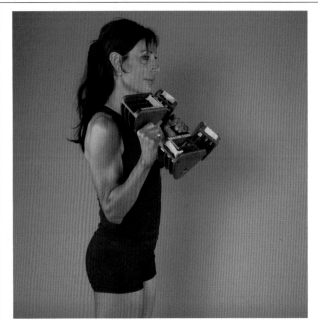

- Continue lifting dumbbells to your shoulders by contracting your biceps.

- Keep palms facing each other throughout the movement and elbows tucked to the sides of your body.

- Lower dumbbells slowly back to start position.

- Elbows do not move. Any swinging or momentum is cheating.

CONCENTRATION CURL, TONERS

Unilateral work involves doing the dynamic portion of the movement one limb at a time

Concentration is an art. It is often associated with focus, discipline, willpower, and connecting with our subconscious. Applying concentration to tasks at hand can take our untapped talents and abilities to another level. During exercise, especially a biceps concentration curl, it is easy to get distracted and let the mind wander. Your full attention is needed.

During an isometric action, when you are contracting a muscle without any other movement, you have the ability to recruit more muscle fibers. This is because at low muscular demands, your body recruits slow-twitch muscle fibers. With greater intensity and effort, the fast-twitch fibers are activated.

Your body is made up of both slow-twitch and fast-twitch

Concentration Curl Start

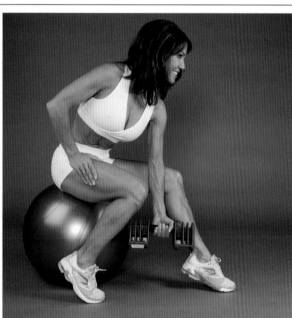

- Sit on ball, legs apart, neutral spine. Retract shoulders and engage abdominals.

- Bend over and with your left hand grasp the dumbbell between your feet, palm up, allowing the dumbbell to hang toward the floor.

- Press the back of the left upper arm firmly on the left inner thigh. Maintain alignment of upper and lower arm.

Concentration Curl Finish

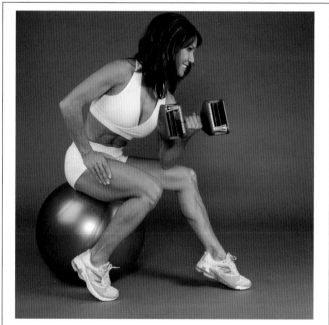

- Slowly curl the dumbbell up by contracting your biceps throughout the movement. Give an extra squeeze when the dumbbell reaches your shoulder.

- Lower the dumbbell until your arm is fully extended. Remain bent over the entire time.

- Repeat with other arm.

muscle fibers. Fast-twitch fibers have larger diameters than slow-twitch fibers and can generally produce more force, or strength. Slow-twitch fibers are more resistant to fatigue and are beneficial to your endurance goals.

Your individual and predominant muscle-fiber type is a combination of genetics and training. Slow-twitch folk (think shaped like a beanpole) should increase weight, minimize reps, and rest longer. Fast-twitch individuals (think track sprinter) should do more reps and rest less between sets.

Elastic Toner Curl Start

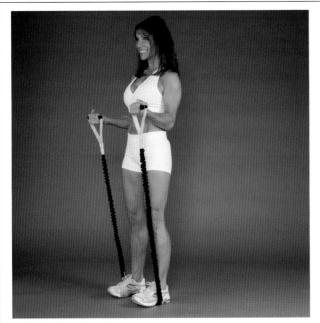

- Place toner under both feet and center the handles. Ensure tension is tight by pre-stretching.

- Use neutral body position. Engage abdominals and retract shoulders.

- Start with hands at your sides, palms up, elbows tucked tight to sides of the body.

- Curl handles up evenly by contracting your biceps.

Elastic Toner Curl Finish

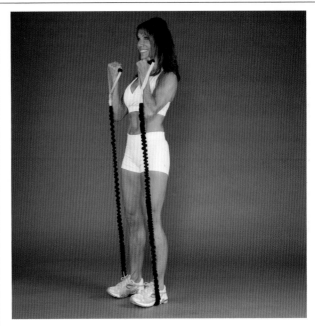

- Continue to curl handles up to shoulder level. Keep elbows at your sides.

- Lower toner slowly back to start position.

- Remember to keep the elastic taut.

BICEPS

87

LYING BICEPS CURL

Full-range-of-motion exercises mimic many real-life scenarios

The biceps brachii is the prominent muscle on the front side of your upper arm. The brachialis is the muscle located on the front of the upper arm, just beneath the biceps, closer to the elbow. Both are responsible for flexing and rotating the elbow and forearm. The biceps, or "guns," are often regarded as symbols of strength. How many times have you seen children and adult men flex this muscle a la Arnold Schwarzenegger to display muscular prowess?

The lying biceps curl is an Arnold staple. When you lie down on a bench for this exercise, the biceps stretch fully at the bottom of the movement and the muscle lengthens. The range of motion is maximized during each lift. Because of the angle, every contraction is a full effort to offset the pull of gravity.

The first thing you will notice when you lie down with weights in your hands is the immediate stretch in your shoul-

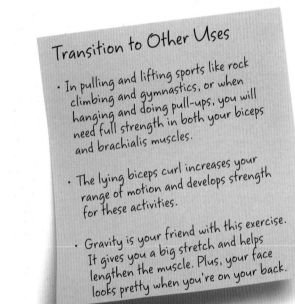

Transition to Other Uses

- In pulling and lifting sports like rock climbing and gymnastics, or when hanging and doing pull-ups, you will need full strength in both your biceps and brachialis muscles.

- The lying biceps curl increases your range of motion and develops strength for these activities.

- Gravity is your friend with this exercise. It gives you a big stretch and helps lengthen the muscle. Plus, your face looks pretty when you're on your back.

Lying Biceps Curl: Position 1

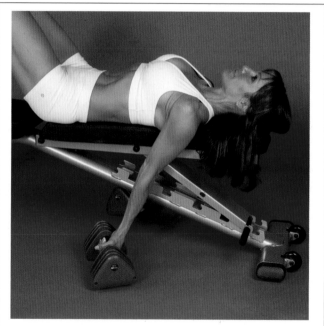

- Select a lighter weight for this exercise than used for upright curls.

- Lie back on the bench, legs together, knees bent, and feet flat on the bench.

- Grab dumbbells with palms up. Dumbbells should hang.

- If needed, add a block under the bench to raise it to accomodate your arms hanging down freely.

ders and arms. This often feels good. It may also be damaging, so proceed with caution. Always start a new exercise with light weights (less than five pounds) and single sets (between eight and ten reps) to see how your body responds. Add this exercise to your routine at least twice a month to achieve its benefits.

Lying Biceps Curl: Position 2

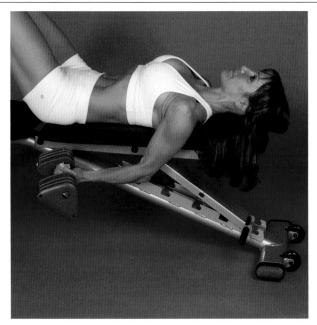

- Curl the dumbbells slowly.

- Keep your upper arms and elbows still, only moving your lower arms.

- This exercise is one of the best stretch and contraction moves for biceps.

Lying Biceps Curl: Position 3

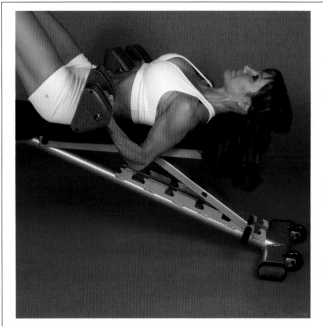

- Continue to curl the dumbbells to your shoulders.

- Lower the dumbbells back toward the floor, resisting the weight all the way down.

- Variation: Lift your head off the bench and look down over your chest during the movement.

BICEPS

PREACHER CURL, WRIST CURL

This exercise is called a preacher curl because if done correctly, it looks like you're praying

A preacher curl is typically done using a special bench. If you are not training at a gym and need an alternate resource, grab a firmly inflated stability ball.

The preacher curl targets a specific part of the biceps muscle and helps fill in the space between the lower biceps and the elbow joint.

Position your body against the bench or ball and extend your arm over the top. Additional stress is transferred to the lower muscle from this extended arm angle. If your objective is to create more shape to the biceps muscle, the preacher curl will deliver.

To avoid strength or size imbalance in the arms, the wrists

Preacher Curl Start

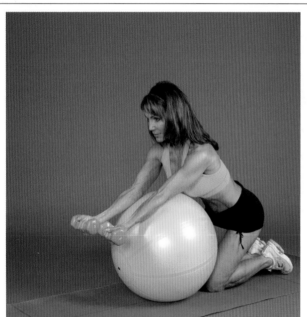

- This exercise is typically performed on a specially designed bench, but a stability ball also works.

- Kneel with the ball in front of you and grasp dumbbells with your palms up.

- Place the back of your arms on the ball. Adjust kneeling position so armpits rest near the top of the ball.

Preacher Curl Finish

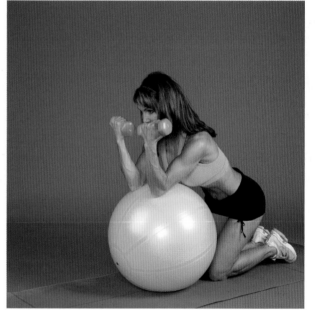

- Curl dumbbells by contracting your biceps. The back of your upper arms remain on the ball.

- Lower dumbbells until arm is fully extended.

- Variations: Elbows closer together targets outer biceps. Elbows farther apart works inner biceps. Also try one arm at a time.

must be exercised. Dumbbells are better for training this body part than a bar, because they provide isolateral training, allowing your forearms to work independently.

Reverse wrist curls isolate the muscles on top of the forearm. The range of motion is limited during this movement, so don't be alarmed if you can't execute the move as much as the underhand curl. The forearms are primarily made up of slow-twitch muscle fibers, which are associated with endurance, so aim for high repetitions (12 to 15) during a training session.

Reverse Wrist Curl Start

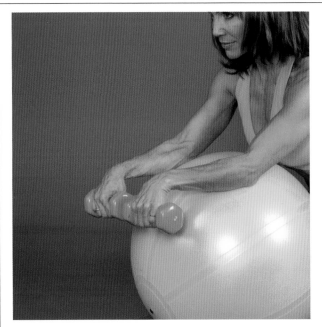

- Kneel with the stability ball in front of you. Grasp dumbbells with your palms down.

- Rest forearms on the ball so wrists are just beyond the surface and can move freely without hitting the ball.

- Start by dropping your wrists, pointing your knuckles down.

Reverse Wrist Curl Finish

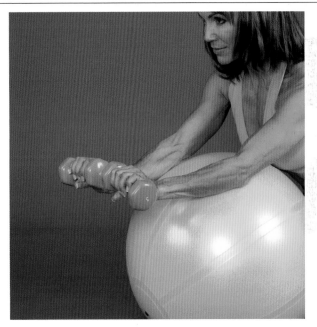

- Hyperextend your wrists up as high as possible without moving forearms.

- Keep your elbows at wrist height through full range of motion. This maintains resistance.

- Return until wrists are fully flexed.

- Variations: Use flat bench instead of ball. Try one arm at a time, resting forearm on thigh while seated.

BICEPS

PLIÉ CURL WITH ROTATION

A comprehensive movement that involves the biceps, core, and lower body will burn more calories

Still wondering if you're going to build big biceps? Feeling apprehensive when it comes to training the biceps muscles in a "manly" fashion? Here's an exercise that will appeal to your feminine senses. Practiced by Sana Bridges, Pilates instructor and our svelte over-50 model, the plié curl with rotation creates cooperative movement throughout the body.

The options for training your biceps are many. When you sit, stand, squat, lie down, balance, add rotation, and use single arm movement, the dynamics change. In brief, any new challenge to the muscle creates an adaptation response that ultimately delivers positive results.

During a plié curl with rotation, you use half of your range

Plié Curl: Position 1

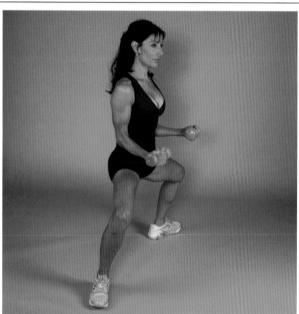

- Use an extra-wide stance with toes turned out at a comfortable angle and knees aligned with toes. Lower into a squat position.

- Find neutral spine, retract shoulders, and engage abdominals.

- Hold lightweight dumbbells with palms up, forearms parallel to the floor. Tuck your elbows tight to the body.

Plié Curl: Position 2

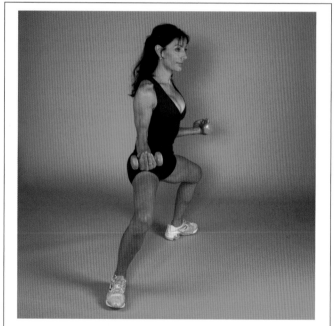

- Maintain plié squat position and keep upper body still.

- Keeping forearms parallel to the floor, move hands out to the sides, rotating at your shoulders.

- Keep elbows tucked at your sides during rotation.

of motion, which demands greater control. This small movement has similar benefits to a popular biceps exercise called twenty-ones. Twenty-ones are when you curl the weight 7 times from bottom to mid range, 7 times from mid range to top, and 7 times for a full curl.

The plié curl with rotation is a compound exercise that also works the core and lower body. The basic ballet plié turns out the legs and develops the tendons and muscles of the thighs, calves, ankles, and feet. As your knees bend, a slight counterpull upward develops the buttocks, thighs, and abdomen.

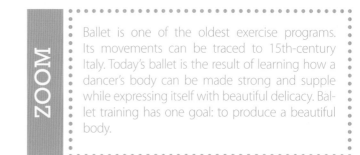
Plié Curl: Position 3

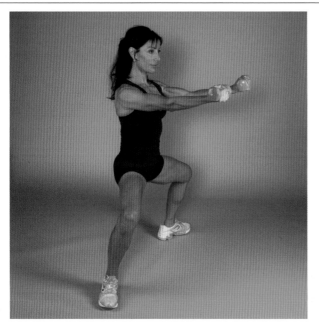

- Maintain plié squat position and keep upper body still.

- Extend arms out in front of the body, maintaining a palms-up grip on the dumbbells. Entire arms are now parallel to the floor.

- Avoid locking your elbows. Maintain natural bend.

Plié Curl: Position 4

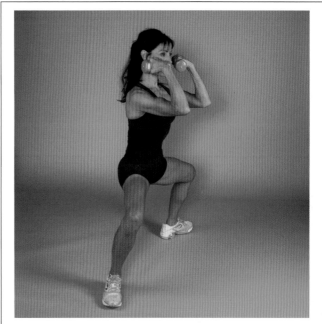

- Maintain plié squat position and keep upper body still.

- Keeping upper arms parallel to the floor, curl the dumbbells above your shoulders.

- Squeeze your biceps.

- Return arms to the start position with elbows tucked tight to the body and forearms parallel to the floor.

BICEPS

93

NARROW PUSH-UP, DIPS
These exercises are deceptively simple looking, yet when performed properly, they are hard to master

The triceps, or triceps brachii muscle, is the large muscle on the back of your upper arm. It accounts for about 20 percent of your upper arm muscle mass and is responsible for extension of the elbow joint, or the straightening of the arm. The antagonist, or oppositional muscle, is the biceps. It is important to maintain balance between the triceps and biceps for muscular balance and effectiveness.

To train the triceps, you can incorporate a combination of isolation and compound movements. Dips and narrow push-ups are both compound pressing exercises and popular methods for training the triceps in that they can be performed anywhere, anytime.

Narrow Push-up Start

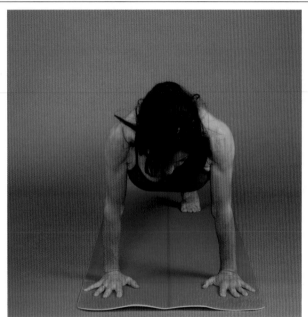

- Assume the plank position with shoulders over wrists. Maintain neutral body position in one straight line.

- Lift your right leg off the mat, extending it until it is even with your shoulders.

Narrow Push-up Finish

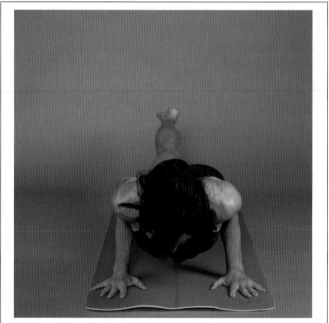

- Maintain straight body alignment and lifted right leg.

- Bend your elbows, keeping upper arms hugged into your sides.

- Lower your body toward

the floor until elbows make a right angle.

- Push back into your left heel.

- For easier options, keep both feet on the mat or drop your knees to the floor.

Narrow push-ups focus on the triceps, minimizing chest and shoulder involvement. Yoga students make the narrow push-up, called *chaturanga*, or four limbs, look idyllic. Practice this posture with your elbows in, shoulder blades retracted, and torso parallel to the floor.

A seated dip is a perfect starting place if you are at a beginner or intermediate training level. Using a bench, or a chair, place your hands behind you on the edge, shoulder-width apart. Extend your legs in front of you, changing the level of difficulty by placing them more underneath you or extending them far-

ther out. When ready to start the activity, slide your body so that your bottom is suspended in the air as close to the bench as possible. Weight distribution will depend on where you've placed your feet. Slowly lower your bottom, keeping it close to the bench, and imagine sitting down on the floor. Press up again to a full arm extended position.

Both of these exercises may aggravate chronic shoulder pain. If you suffer from a shoulder-joint ailment such that these exercises are painful, move on to other triceps exercises in this chapter.

Bench Dip

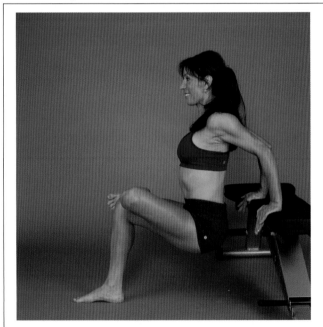

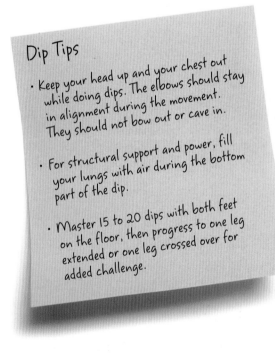

Dip Tips

- Keep your head up and your chest out while doing dips. The elbows should stay in alignment during the movement. They should not bow out or cave in.

- For structural support and power, fill your lungs with air during the bottom part of the dip.

- Master 15 to 20 dips with both feet on the floor, then progress to one leg extended or one leg crossed over for added challenge.

- Sit on the bench and cross left foot over right knee. Fully extend arms shoulder-width apart, palms on the edge of the bench.

- Slide your buttocks off the bench so arms are supporting your weight.

- Bend elbows, lowering your body to mimic a sitting position. Push back up to start.

KICKBACK

The kickback is an isolation exercise; movement is restricted to one joint and one muscle group

The purpose of the kickback is to build strength and tone the triceps, with the goal of making any flabby bits go away. While this move will indeed help the character of the muscle, it will not give you the cut look that you are after until you lose body fat. Consider your program an unveiling. If you start defining your muscles now, when you do lose weight,

you'll see the sexy shape you want.

It takes effort to make changes. Lifting weights that are too light will not get you there. Kickbacks, however, need a weight amount that errs on the side of light instead of heavy. Your chosen weight for kickbacks should allow you to successfully lift between 12 and 15 reps with good form. You

One-Arm Kickback Start

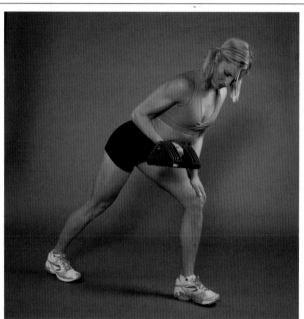

One-Arm Kickback Finish

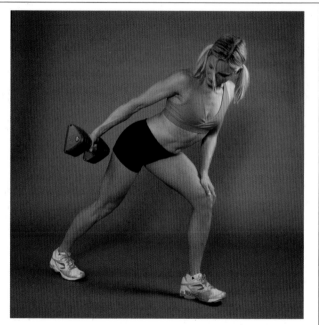

- Grab the dumbbell in your right hand, palm up. While maintaining neutral body position, lunge your right leg back.

- Keep upper arm tucked against your side and your elbow at a 90-degree angle.

- Your upper arm and leg should be in alignment.

- Slowly extend your lower arm back by contracting the triceps. Keep upper arm at your side.

- Slowly lower the dumbbell to the start position,

being mindful not to bend your elbow more than 90 degrees so that you keep constant tension in the muscle.

- Repeat with the left arm.

should feel fatigue during the last couple of kickbacks with every set.

Controlled motion is key. If you allow the arm to swing at all, you will lose the isolating benefits of the kickback. Hand position for a kickback varies. The hammer position is the most popular for developing the upper area of the triceps muscle. This position is comfortable and the grip is less cumbersome. Turning the palms up and dangling the wrist a bit will add resistance, increasing the challenge and difficulty.

ZOOM

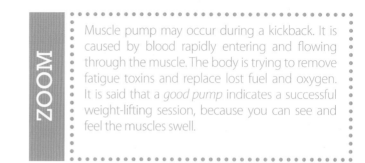

Muscle pump may occur during a kickback. It is caused by blood rapidly entering and flowing through the muscle. The body is trying to remove fatigue toxins and replace lost fuel and oxygen. It is said that a *good pump* indicates a successful weight-lifting session, because you can see and feel the muscles swell.

Kickback Start

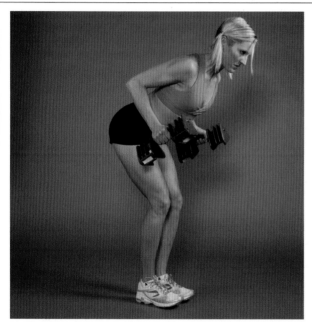

- These are also called triceps extensions.

- Grab dumbbells with both hands, palms facing each other (hammer position).

- Maintain neutral spine and keep your legs together. Bend your knees and bend forward slightly.

- Keep upper arms tucked against your sides and elbows at a 90-degree angle.

Kickback Finish

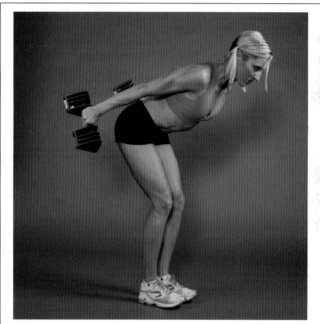

- Without moving your body, slowly extend your lower arms back by contracting the triceps. Keep upper arms at your sides.

- Head forward, neutral spine, abdominals engaged.

- Avoid the temptation to swing the dumbbells. Any momentum diminishes the effectiveness of the exercise.

TRICEPS

OVERHEAD EXTENSION

Fully extend your arms at the end of these exercises to develop your triceps muscle

The overhead extension, or standing triceps extension, is regarded as one of the best exercises to build the full sweep of the triceps muscle. Naturally when many women hear the word *build*, they panic. Allow a moment for review, because this point about building muscle mass cannot be emphasized enough.

Women who are training specifically to build muscles of herculean proportions may, after extensive training, develop muscles that adopt this description. It is rare to see a woman with a horseshoe-shaped, bulging triceps muscle. It also takes specific training, often coupled with hormonal therapy, to achieve these results.

Overhead Extension Start

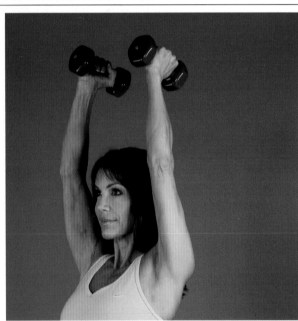

Overhead Extension Finish

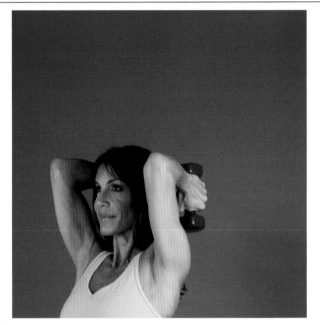

- Stand with neutral body position, legs together and feet shoulder-width apart.

- Grab dumbbells with both hands, palms facing each other.

- Retract shoulders and engage abdominals. Raise arms straight overhead with dumbbells in hammer position.

- Keep a slight bend in your elbows.

- Maintaining neutral body position, lower forearms behind your head while keeping your upper arms still.

- Flex your wrists at the bottom to avoid hitting the

dumbbells on the back of your neck.

- Keep elbows shoulder-width apart and wrists close together.

98

Body type is one of several genetic factors. Body types are classified as mesomorphs, who are muscular; endomorphs, who are more rounded and voluptuous; and ectomorphs, who are slim and linear shaped. Mesomorphs respond to strength training by building muscle mass faster than ectomorphs, even when they follow the same routine. Endomorphs generally need to lose body fat before they see muscle definition. Ectomorphs have more of a challenge in building muscle mass, even when they try to do so.

The golden rule applies for training the triceps, and lifting weights in general. If you want to get stronger, lift heavier weights with fewer repetitions. If you want to increase endurance, use adequate weights and more reps. Adequate weight means you can perform approximately 12 to 15 reps of a given exercise during one set before failure.

The two-arm triceps extension and the seated triceps extension can be performed with a bar or dumbbells. Standing, sitting, or lying positions are common for each. When doing single-arm versions lying down, the dumbbell will cross over the face, not behind the head. These are called *skull crushers*.

One-Arm Overhead Extension Start

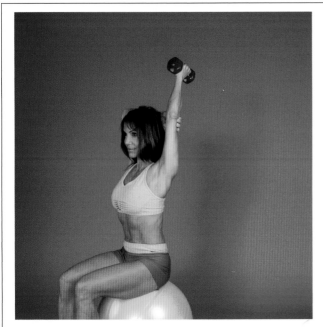

- Sit on the ball with neutral spine. Grab a dumbbell with the left hand, palm in.

- Raise left arm straight overhead. Support your left elbow by grabbing it with your right hand behind your head.

One-Arm Overhead Extension Finish

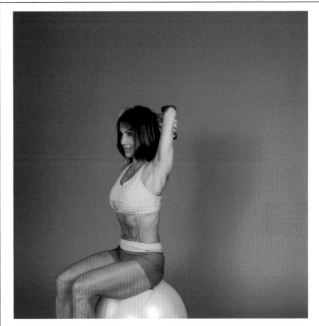

- Maintaining neutral spine, lower the dumbbell behind your head to the base of your neck while keeping your upper arm still. The dumbbells will travel in a diagonal motion.

- Avoid arching your back when lowering the dumbbell behind your head.

- Repeat with other arm.

TRI LIFT AND TAP

Positive affirmations affect your subconscious; they make your muscles stronger and more active

The tri lift and tap is another Sana Bridges specialty exercise that incorporates functional movement into a triceps routine. It adds elements of flexibility, core stability, lower-body strength, and precision.

This exercise starts out resembling a traditional triceps bent-over, two-arm kickback. Choose a small, lightweight dumbbell for this exercise; a large round-plate dumbbell is too large to properly finish the move. During the second and third phase of this exercise, the dumbbell is positioned behind your back, which is in and of itself a challenge for most. After the tap behind your back, you will lift the dumbbells higher, creating more space between your body and arms.

Tri Lift and Tap: Position 1

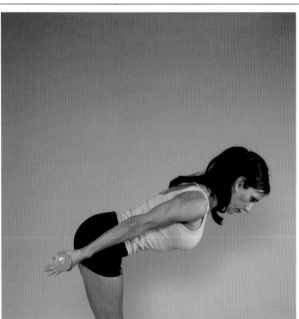

- Use standing neutral body position with legs together.

- Hold dumbbells by your sides, palms back. Retract your shoulders and engage abdominals.

- Bend forward from your hips until your upper body is almost parallel to the floor.

- Keep arms at your sides.

Tri Lift and Tap: Position 2

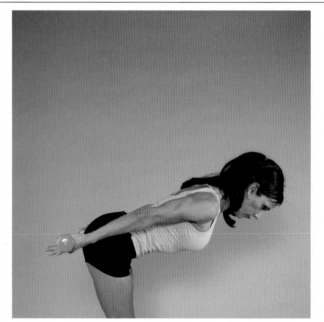

- Maintain neutral spine and keep your neck aligned with your back.

- With dumbbells resting in your palms and arms

straight, lift your arms up so they are perfectly parallel with your back.

- If needed, bend your knees to accommodate.

In addition to activating the shoulders, triceps, and core, the tri lift and tap improves your hamstring flexibility and lower-body strength. Keep your legs together and slightly bend your knees, keeping your weight balanced on your heels and balls of your feet. For maximum conditioning, your back should be parallel to the floor during the entire movement.

If you are inflexible, it is acceptable to modify the move by not bending over to a parallel position. There will always be a creative means to accommodate your limitations. Just make sure you honor neutral body position (good form).

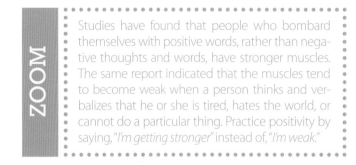
Tri Lift and Tap: Position 3

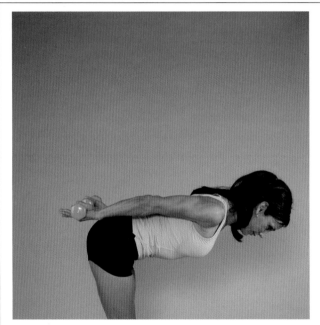

- Continue to maintain strict body position.

- With dumbbells resting in your palms and your arms straight, lift over top of buttocks and tap dumbbells together.

- Avoid bending your elbows as much as possible or dropping your chest down.

Tri Lift and Tap: Position 4

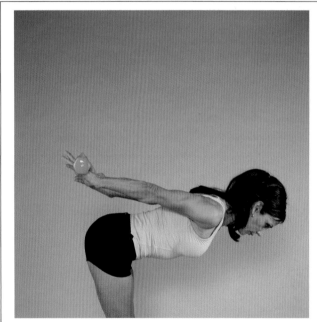

- Release tap and keep arms at shoulder width.

- With arms straight, lift your arms and dumbbells higher above your back.

- Feel free to stand in between reps to rest your back.

TRICEPS

PRESS-DOWN

Triceps exercises increase strength, tone, and muscular development to the upper arm

The triceps press-down is an isolation exercise performed on a cable system or with elastic toners. If using a cable pulley system at the gym, attach a rope, or a short bar (V handle, flat or bent), overhead to the carabiner. At home, anchor the elastic toner to the top of a door frame.

The triceps press-down delivers continuous tension dur-

ing the exercise. This progressive resistance stimulates the muscle growth. The exercise targets the triceps through a full range of motion. With a rope, or elastic toner, you can add a twist at the end of the press, rotating your thumbs in toward your body, for more activation of muscle fibers.

In order to target the lateral and long heads of the triceps—

Press-Down Start

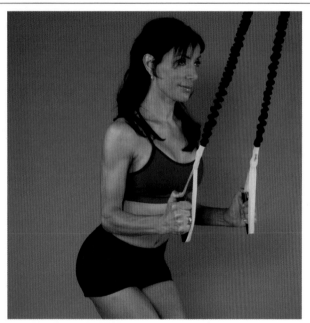

- Anchor the toner overhead. Stand facing the anchor and grab both handles with palms facing each other.

- Retract shoulders, engage abdominals, bend knees, and lean forward slightly.

- Keep elbows tucked to your sides at a 90-degree angle.

- Start with tension on the elastic.

Press-Down Finish

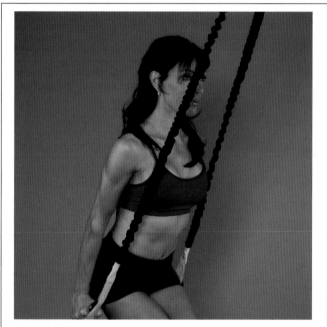

- Maintaining body position, press the handles down by contracting your triceps.

- Squeeze your muscles through full extension, until arms are parallel to your body.

- Return to start.

- Variation: Rotate your hand at the bottom of the move, pronating (palms back), and pull handles slightly apart.

102

the horseshoe-shaped muscle—grab a small handle for the one-arm, reverse-grip press-down (not shown). For this variation, you should stand at an angle to the toner so that your working arm is in line with the cord. Place your hand through the handle, palm up, and begin the movement.

Whether you are standing or using the bent-over variation, it is important to keep your back in neutral body position, including your core engaged. Any deviation will lessen the effectiveness of the exercise.

Bent-Over Press-Down Start

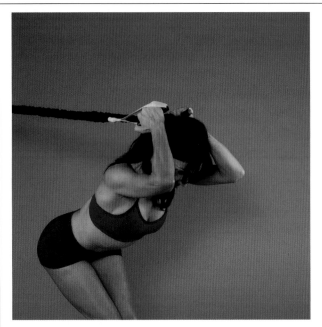

- Anchor the toner at chest level. Stand facing away from the anchor.

- Grab both handles overhead with palms facing each other. Bend forward until upper body is almost parallel to the floor.

- Raise arms overhead, elbows at a 90-degree angle and tucked near your ears.

- Start with tension on the toner.

Bent-Over Press-Down Finish

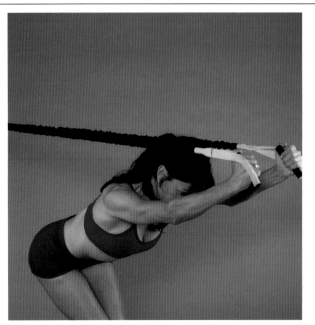

- Extend arms overhead by contracting your triceps. Arms should be aligned with torso. Keep palms facing each other.

- Return to start.

- Allowing your back to over-arch or hips to move can lessen the effectiveness of the exercise.

TRICEPS

103

INTERNAL, EXTERNAL ROTATION

The shoulder is the most mobile joint in the body and requires stabilizer-muscle strength

Rotator cuff is a collective term that refers to several muscles in your shoulder. Comprised of four small muscles called the subscapularis, infraspinatus, supraspinatus, and teres minor, the rotator cuff has the greatest range of motion of any joint in your body. These muscles and the tendons that attach the muscles to the bone connect your upper arm to your shoul-

der blade and keep the ball of your upper arm in its socket. Your shoulder health depends on these muscles!

We use our rotator cuffs so often in daily activities that involve one-sided and overhead movements, like lifting, pushing, pulling, pressing, holding, stirring, and even sweeping, that the little muscles just can't keep up with our repetitive

Internal Rotation Start

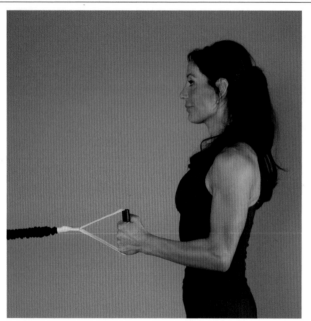

- Anchor the elastic toner at elbow height. Stand facing the anchor.

- Grasp handle with your left hand, palm in. Fix elbow to your side.

- Maintain neutral body position. Retract your shoulders, engage your abdominals.

Internal Rotation Finish

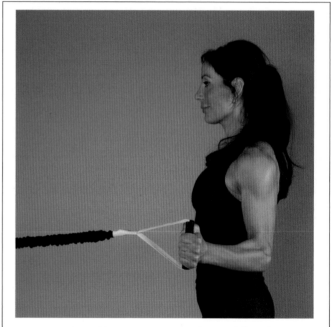

- Maintain neutral body position.

- Keeping elbow bent and fixed to the left side of your waist, rotate lower arm out to side. Initiate the movement with your shoulder.

- Stay at midline of the body.

- Keep tension in the toner throughout the movement.

- Repeat with the other arm.

demands. They need proper strength training to keep them fit and able to perform the daily tasks. Otherwise, injury may ensue.

A rotator cuff injury can be an irritation that may go away, an inflammation without permanent damage, or tendinitis, which is a complete or partial tear of the muscle. None are pleasant. Preventive medicine in the form of exercise takes just a few minutes.

The elastic toner is your ally here. A responsible and practical idea is to anchor the toner to a point near your office desk, or some other place where it is easily accessible. Make a commitment to train both the external and internal rotator cuff three times per week. Perform 15 to 20 reps and three sets each.

Always stretch after training the rotators. Door stretching is recommended. Try grabbing the knob with both hands, straightening your arms, bending forward, and leaning back/down. Then, put both outstretched arms high, with the elbows at 90 degrees (field goal position) on each side of the door frame and lean in to it.

External Rotation Start

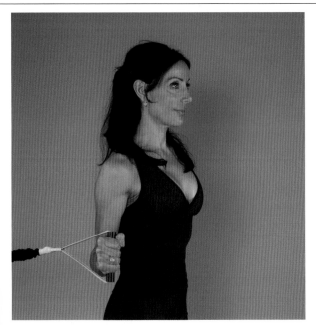

- Anchor the elastic toner at elbow height. Stand facing away from the anchor.

- Grasp the handle with your right hand, palm in. Fix your elbow to your side.

- Assume neutral body position. Retract your shoulders, engage your abdominals.

External Rotation Finish

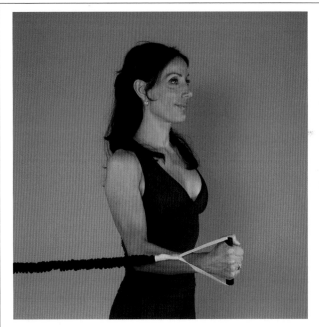

- Maintain neutral body position.

- Keeping elbow bent and fixed to the right side of your waist, rotate lower arm across your body at midline.

- Initiate the movement with your shoulder.

- Hand should finish near your left rib cage.

- Repeat with other arm.

SCAPULAR STABILIZATION
The shoulder blade helps the rotator cuff to stabilize the shoulder while in motion

The scapula, also called the shoulder blade or shoulder girdle, connects your arm to your collarbone. It's that flat, triangular bone that pokes out on the back, visible in children and skinny folk. The scapula helps the rotator cuff stabilize the shoulder joint while in motion. If the shoulder blade is unstable, too much pressure is placed on the rotator cuff and problems arise.

Weak stabilizers will prevent you from lifting heavy weights, even if your big muscles are capable. The more stabilizers and synergists you work, the more muscle fibers you stimulate.

Here are some strengthening exercises for the muscles that support the scapula:

Incorrect Scapular Stabilization

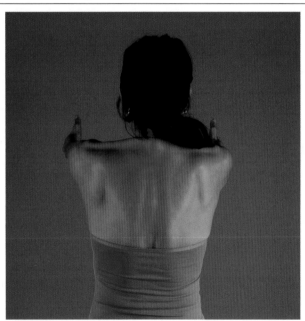

- Lifting the shoulders and rounding the back is poor form. This protraction posture compromises the shoulders and spine and increases the risk for injury.

- Incorrect posture, lack of flexibility, and improper training can cause tense shoulders and neck ache.

Correct Scapular Stabilization

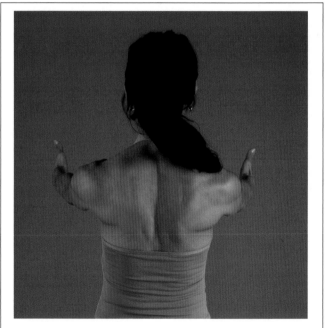

- Retracting the shoulders involves multiple movements. Start by lengthening your spine and holding your head high. Pull your shoulders backwards, as if you are placing them down and into your back pockets. Don't just pinch them together.

- Your shoulders should be low and under your ears.

Shoulder roll – Stand with arms at sides. Move shoulders forward, shrug up, move backward, squeeze blades together, pull down. Repeat five times and reverse direction.

Supine shoulder lift – Lie on back. Raise arms straight up. Lift until shoulder blade is off the floor. Return and repeat ten times. Add light dumbbell as strength increases.

Prone shoulder lift – Lie on belly. Hold light dumbbell with both hands. Place over lower back, palms up. Lift away from back. Repeat ten times.

Incorrect Overhead Stabilization

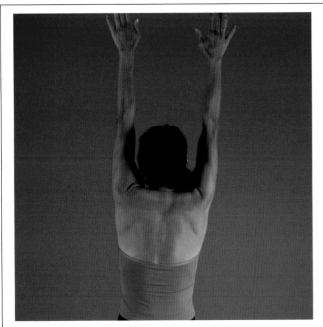

- When reaching up (also called elevation), practice mindful movement and avoid lifting your shoulders. Poor form compromises your shoulder joint, impinges the neck, and overworks the traps.

- Beautiful muscular development will not happen with poor form.

Correct Overhead Stabilization

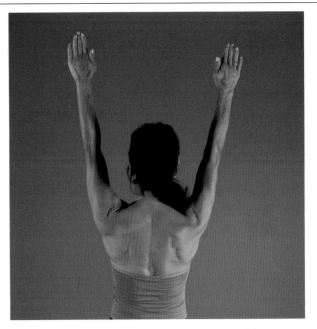

- The muscles in your back (lats) should be the primary movers when you raise your hands overhead.

- Keeping your shoulder blades (scapula) pulled down, also called depression, helps stabilize your shoulders and prepare you for lifting.

- Learn to sit, walk, and stand using proper scapular stabilization for improved posture.

SHOULDERS

SHOULDER PRESS, DECLINE PUSH-UP

Decline push-ups are very difficult and should be attempted only by physically fit individuals

Deltoids (delts) have three heads that are responsible for different actions. The medial or lateral deltoids help you raise your arms up to the sides. The anterior or front deltoids allow you to raise your arms straight up in front of you. The posterior or rear deltoids make it possible for you to move your arms toward your back at shoulder level.

Your trapezius muscles (traps) are technically part of your shoulders and upper-back muscles. The top part, which is at the top of the shoulders and the base of your neck, is responsible for scapular elevation or shrugging.

Strengthening your shoulders has several benefits beyond increased performance and upper-body strength. Because

Shoulder Press Start

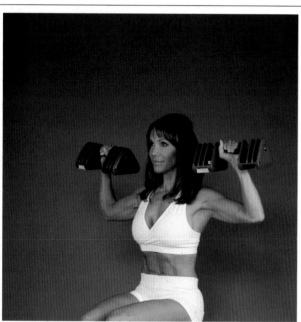

- The shoulder press is also known as the Military Press

- Sit on a stability ball with neutral body position. Keep legs together and feet planted on the floor.

- Bring dumbbells over your shoulders with elbows out to your sides and palms forward.

- Retract your shoulders, engage your abdominals.

Shoulder Press Finish

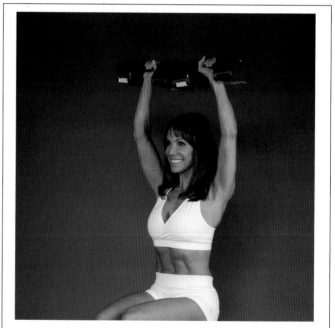

- Keeping elbows out to your sides and aligned with your torso, press dumbbells overhead.

- Continue retracting your shoulders and avoid locking your elbows.

- The front delts are the primary movers; medial delts, traps, and triceps are the secondary movers.

- Variations: Stand. Sit on a bench. Alternate arms.

the shoulders are so susceptible to damage, injury prevention is another benefit. Also, toned well-shaped shoulders make every woman look more fit and put together.

The medial deltoids get the least work during strength training and need isolation exercises. The front and rear delts work a lot during other movements, such as assisting with push-pull exercises like push-ups, chest press, and back work. Inverted push-ups, however, target the desired medial head more than a traditional push-up does.

Decline Push-up Start

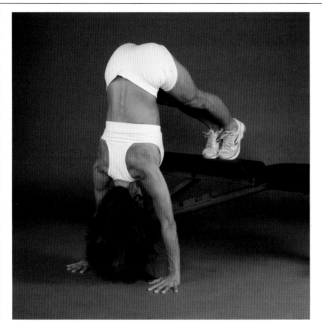

- This is an advanced move. If you're pregnant and/or have certain medical conditions, consult your doctor before performing any inverted exercise.

- Plant hands on the floor, slightly wider than shoulder width; elbows out to your sides.

- Place the balls of your feet on a bench and extend legs.

Decline Push-up Finish

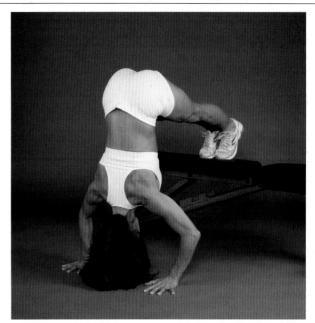

- Retract shoulders and engage abdominals.

- Bend elbows to slowly lower your body. Resist gravity by controlling the movement. Do not touch your head to the floor.

- Keeping your spine neutral and upper body vertical will keep focus on your shoulders and triceps, not your chest.

SHOULDERS

LATERAL SIDE RAISE

Train the sides of your shoulders with isolated movements to create a sexy, shaped muscle

In order to give your shoulders a full, round, shapely look, you must isolate the medial head of the deltoid with specific exercise. This muscle runs down the side of the arm and provides a sinewy curve that makes wearing short-sleeve shirts desirable. The lateral side raise is one of the best exercises to train this body part.

Before you pick up dumbbells or elastic toners and start this exercise, understand that lateral side raises can be demanding on the rotator cuff. They can compress the area and cause impingement-like symptoms, resulting in an ache or pain. To further the complexity of the situation, the shoulder—comprised of three joints: the sternoclavicular, acromioclavicular,

Lateral Side Raise Start

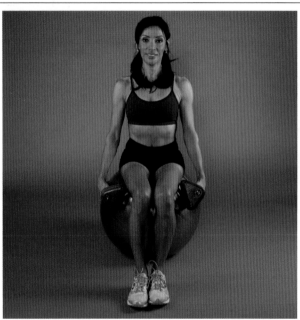

- Grab dumbbells with palms facing each other. Sit on a ball with neutral body position.

- Walk feet forward until you're seated on the edge of the ball. Lean your upper

body forward slightly; legs together, feet planted on the floor.

- Allow dumbbells to hang naturally at your sides.

Lateral Side Raise Finish

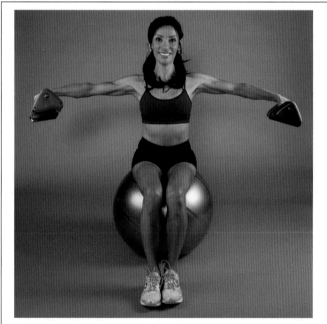

- Retract shoulders and engage abdominals.

- With elbows slightly bent, raise your upper arms to your sides until your elbows are at shoulder height. Do not hunch your shoulders.

- Maintain fixed elbows and upper body position. Palms will face the floor at the top of the movement.

and the glenohumeral—is stressed during a lateral side raise, and takes on a lot of the workload.

Strengthen your rotator cuff muscles first and employ scapular stabilization exercises before tackling lateral side raises. Lateral side raises engage your forearms and traps during the movement. To maintain focus on the side deltoids, lift your arms only until they are parallel to the floor. Make sure you keep the dumbbell balanced, meaning the back and front end equally high.

Incline Lateral Side Raise

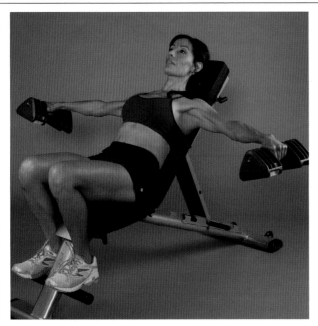

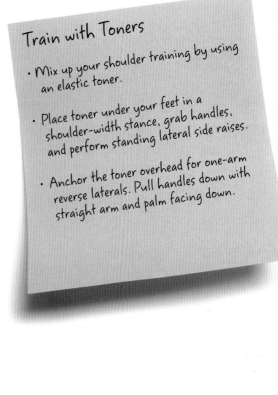

Train with Toners

- Mix up your shoulder training by using an elastic toner.

- Place toner under your feet in a shoulder-width stance, grab handles, and perform standing lateral side raises.

- Anchor the toner overhead for one-arm reverse laterals. Pull handles down with straight arm and palm facing down.

- Adjust bench to incline position. This position also strengthens rotator cuff muscles.

- Use same motion and body position as lateral side raise.

- Medial delt is the primary mover.

- This angle may cause shoulder discomfort. If so, discontinue and try another exercise.

111

FRONT RAISE

Problems occur if your shoulders are so tight that reaching directly overhead is impossible

The front raise exercise targets the anterior deltoid, or front of the shoulder. This muscle is very active in upper-body strength-training routines and needs less isolated training. It is engaged every time you do a pushing exercise, like a chest press or a push-up. It will also try to do the work for the medial (side) delt, which tends to be weaker because of it.

The normal range of motion at the shoulders should allow you to raise your arms above your head without leaning backward, tilting your neck, or scrunching your shoulders. If lifting your arms causes your neck to elevate as well, or your head to tilt forward, you have more stretching and therapeutic exercise to do.

Alternating Front Raise Start

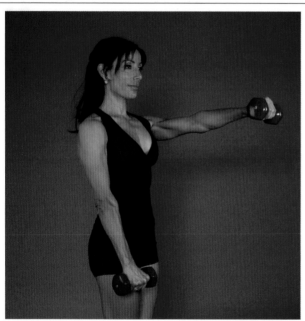

- Grab dumbbells, palms down. Stand with neutral body position.

- Allow the dumbbells to hang in front of your thighs.

- Retract your shoulders and engage your abdominals.

- Use your front delt to lift your left arm in front of your body until it reaches just above shoulder level.

Alternating Front Raise Finish

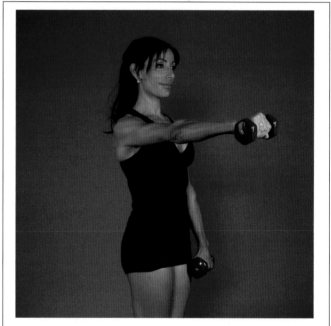

- Maintain a controlled motion, concentrating on the delt.

- Lower the dumbbell back to the front of your thigh and raise right arm using same motion.

- Continue retracting your shoulders and engaging your abdominals to avoid trapezius recruitment.

- Maintain neutral spine and do not arch your lower back to assist.

Front raises improve your range of motion. Choose a seated or standing version. The seated version is stricter, because you cannot use your body to help with the lift. When sitting, use the end of the bench so that the dumbbells in the down position can hang by your sides.

When standing, extend your range by lifting alternating dumbbells above your head in the finish position. The design of your shoulder anatomy allows for this variation, provided you have no contraindications.

Front Raise Push Start

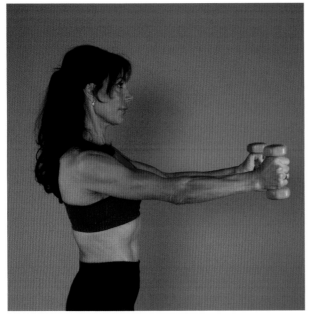

- Grab dumbbells with palms facing each other, arms at your sides.

- Use standing neutral body position, retract your shoulders, and engage your abdominals.

- Raise your arms in front of your body and hold, activating the front delts.

Front Raise Push Finish

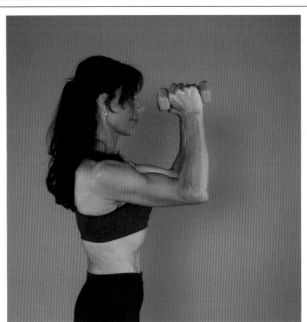

- Maintaining body position, bring heels of hand together in front of you.

- Keep upper arms and elbows stable and bend lower arms to 90 degrees in front of your shoulders.

- Squeeze the dumbbells together and lift your chest while retracting your shoulders.

SHOULDERS

UPRIGHT ROW, SHRUGS

Active in most lifting movements as fixators and stabilizers, the shoulders are often an overstressed muscle

Upright rows and shrug exercises are used as a form of rehabilitation for women who suffer chronic neck-muscle pain. Neck pain, from sitting at a desk and doing monotonous, repetitive tasks, can cause muscular fatigue in the shoulders and neck. The formal name for the malady is *trapezius myalgia*. It causes pain, tension, and trigger points or tight nodules in the skeletal

muscles that when touched can produce tenderness, twitching, and jumping. Physical activity can help fix the problem.

Researchers from Denmark found that participants with pain due to trapezius myalgia achieved at least 70 percent pain reduction by exercising the trapezius muscle. If this works for rehabilitation, it will work for prevention.

Upright Row Start

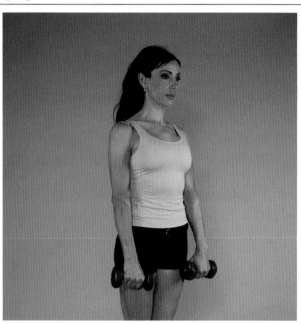

- Grab dumbbells with your palms back. Stand with neutral body position.

- Allow dumbbells to hang in front of your thighs, shoulder-width apart.

- Retract your shoulders and engage your abdominals.

Upright Row Finish

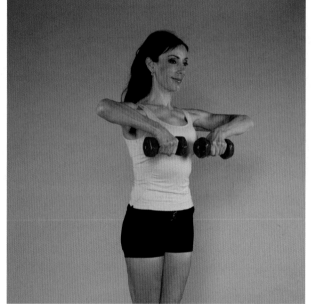

- Bend elbows to pull dumbbells straight up until nearly even with your chest.

- Keep elbows out to sides and aligned with your body. Dumbbells should skim

your body during the lift and release.

- Performing this exercise with dumbbells instead of a bar is easier on the wrists.

Exercises that activate the muscles in the neck and shoulders include shoulder shrugs and upright rows, along with one-arm rows, reverse flies, and lateral raises. The shoulders/deltoids are active in almost every upper body lifting movement. If not the primary, active mover muscle, they are synergists, or fixators.

Fixators keep your bones and joints in a secure position and prevent unnecessary movement of other muscles and stabilizers. This helps you to maintain alignment through a movement and provides balance.

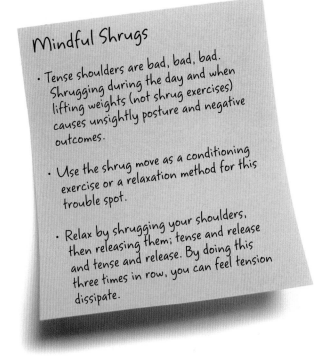

Mindful Shrugs

- Tense shoulders are bad, bad, bad. Shrugging during the day and when lifting weights (not shrug exercises) causes unsightly posture and negative outcomes.

- Use the shrug move as a conditioning exercise or a relaxation method for this trouble spot.

- Relax by shrugging your shoulders, then releasing them; tense and release and tense and release. By doing this three times in row, you can feel tension dissipate.

•••••••••••••••••• RED ● LIGHT ••••••••••••••

If your shoulder and neck problems are from lifting weights, the reasons may be attributed to using incorrect form, changing your exercise routine, overloading your muscles with too much weight, or shoulder impingement problems known as "bursitis." Seek medical attention for proper diagnosis and treatment if you experience swelling, tenderness, stiffness, or pain when lifting and lowering weights.

Incorrect Shrug Position

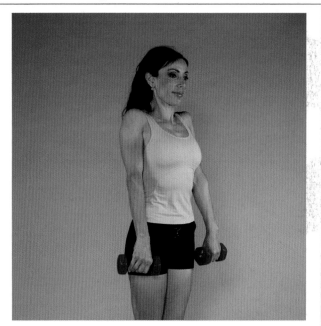

- Poor form is evident by the tension in the neck flexor muscles and the pinching together of the shoulders at the top of the move.

- Raise shoulders straight up, keeping shoulder blades retracted. Do not round your upper back or squeeze your shoulders to your ears.

SHOULDERS

BENT-OVER FLY, CIRCLES

Arm circles strengthen the shoulders and relax them, offering tension relief to the upper back

The reverse fly is recommended to help relieve neck and shoulder pain because it activates the trapezius muscle. It is an exercise that targets the rear delts. The rear delts get a lot of action and indirect work from other strength-training pull exercises, like rows, pull-ups, and pull-downs. Training your rear delts independently helps to improve your posture gen-

erally. If you have weak rear delts, train them independently and make them a priority on your upper-body workout day.

Your hand position changes the focus of the targeted muscle slightly. A *thumbs-down* position focuses almost exclusively on the rear deltoid. A *palms-down* hand position activates the rear deltoids, the traps, the rhomboids, and the

Bent-over Reverse Fly Start

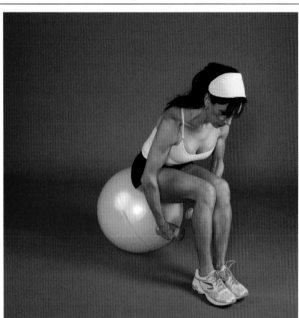

- Grab dumbbells, your palms facing each other. Sit on the edge of the ball with neutral body position. Press legs and feet together.

- Bend forward, pivoting from your hips, so arms

hang down with dumbbells under your knees.

- Do not bend or round the back or collapse midsection into legs.

Bent-over Reverse Fly Finish

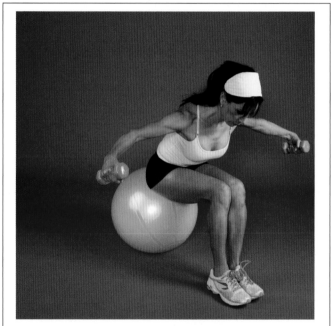

- Retract your shoulders and engage your abdominals.

- Raise arms out to sides to shoulder level by contracting the rear delts. Arms remain in a fixed position with elbows slightly bent.

- Maintain length in neck and lowered shoulders to avoid lifting from the traps.

- Variation: Thumbs-down position.

116

side lats. A *thumbs-up* position is not recommended for this exercise.

Shoulder circles, like rotator-cuff and scapular-stabilization exercises, are other small-muscle exercises that are good to do at the beginning of an exercise session. Circle exercises are done to increase strength and range of motion in the shoulder joint. Circles will open and close the thoracic hinge, which divides the chest and back along the centerline. Variations of shoulder circles include circling upward and backward, forward and downward, and single arm.

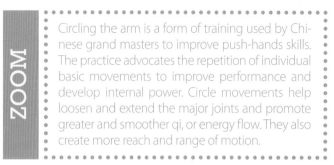

Arm Circles: Position 1

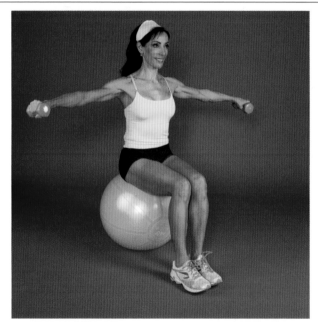

- This exercise may be challenging enough without dumbbells.

- Sit on the ball with neutral spine. Press legs together and plant feet on the floor. Retract your shoulders and engage your abdominals.

- Lift arms to the sides. Keep them straight without hyperextending your elbows.

- Begin circling arms forward, leading from shoulder.

Arm Circles: Position 2

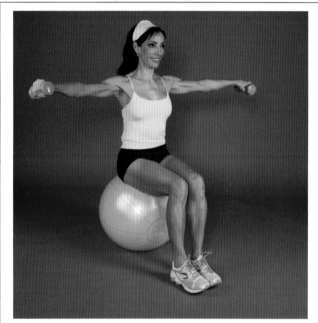

- Maintain body position.

- Reverse the circle direction and continue leading from your shoulders. Use the shoulder blades (scapula) to stabilize the movement.

- Rotate your arms equally. Move to bigger circles as you progress.

- Modifications: Rest on your belly or side and perform one arm movement.

VMO SQUAT
Keeping your knees pain free and functional may be as easy as strengthening your VMO

The vastus medialis oblique (VMO) muscle keeps the kneecap stable and in place. It is a large teardrop-shaped thigh muscle that lies just above and on the inside of the kneecap, or patella. Of the four muscles, collectively called the quadriceps, that make up the front of your thigh, the VMO is the only one that attaches directly to the inner, upper margin of the kneecap.

The VMO muscle can pull inward on the kneecap, while the other three quad muscles pull ever so slightly to the lateral side. If this muscle is weak and untrained, an imbalance occurs. Weakness can manifest itself with knee pain, instability, and abnormal movement of the knee during movement.

Strengthen the VMO and you will increase stability to the

VMO Squat: Position 1

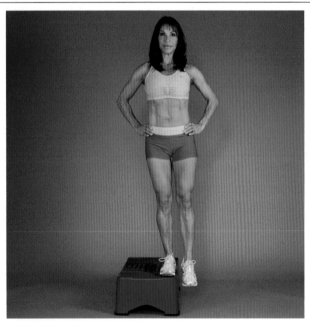

- The knee will always remain behind the toe for this exercise.

- Stand with neutral body position on a stable platform with your hands on your hips.

- Square your hips and balance your weight on your right leg, while left leg dangles to side.

VMO Squat: Position 2

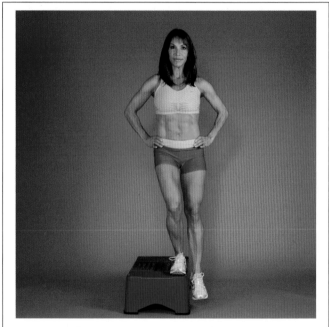

- This is different from a one-leg squat, in that you lean forward into the knee ever so slightly, isolating the vastus medialis.

- Slowly lower your body by bending your right knee, keeping your hips square.

- The left leg should be in alignment with your body.

joint and improve your athletic performance. A common complaint is knee pain. Fitness trainers constantly hear, "I can't do that because my knee hurts." If you don't have an acute injury, chances are you can fix your ache with proper preparation.

If your knees wobble side to side during a squat or step-up despite your best efforts to keep them steady, you are weak in this area. Fix the situation by exercising the VMO.

GREEN ● LIGHT

Strengthen your VMO and its tendons by quad setting. With a straight leg, contract (tense) the muscles in your thigh as hard as you can. Hold for six seconds. Or, perform a quarter-squat. With your back against a wall, squat to a 30 degree knee flexion, then stand straight and contract the quads strongly. Full squats can be a VMO exercise by straightening the knee and tensing the quads every rep.

VMO Squat: Position 3

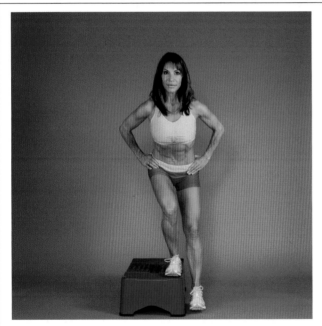

- Maintain body position.

- Continue lowering your body by bending your right knee. Keep upper body as erect as possible.

- Left leg should drop between 8 and 10 inches.

- Your right knee must remain in alignment with your foot and upper leg. Any side-to-side movement is an indication of weakness.

VMO Squat: Position 4

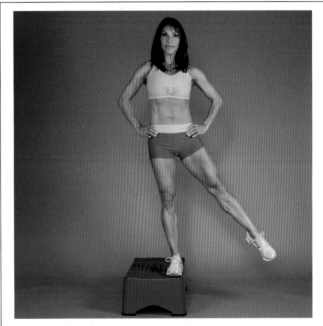

- Adjust the balance of your weight so you're centered on your right foot.

- Press into the step and lift your body up by contracting your VMO.

- When almost standing, extend your left leg to the side, keeping hips square. This targets the gluteus medius, stabilizing the pelvis.

- Repeat with other leg.

FULL SQUAT

The king of all exercises, the squat delivers calorie-burning and muscle-building goodness every time

The squat is the ultimate compound exercise. It tests your legs, core, and functional ability. It builds muscle, burns calories, and delivers more bang for your buck than any other exercise. Because the squat is a dynamic movement that involves bending the knees and stabilizing the low back, proper form is critical.

Review proper form and neutral body position. Perfect your squat technique by using your body weight only, and then progress to dumbbells. Dumbbells can be held at your sides or on your shoulders. Eventually, if you are at a gym and have adequate training and muscular foundation, use an Olympic bar and a squat cage.

Incorrect Squat Position

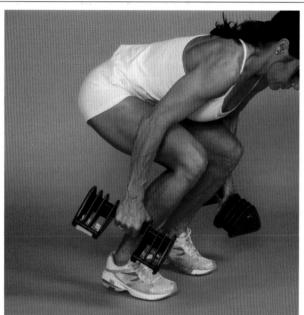

- Performed incorrectly, squats can injure your back and knees.

- If you can't see your toes because your knees are blocking them, it is a sign of bad form.

- Bad form includes bent upper body, with weight on toes; rounded back; protruding abdominals; and arms holding the weight out of the vertical plane.

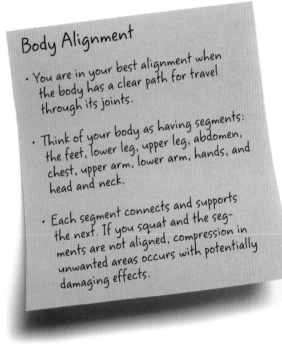

Body Alignment

- You are in your best alignment when the body has a clear path for travel through its joints.

- Think of your body as having segments: the feet, lower leg, upper leg, abdomen, chest, upper arm, lower arm, hands, and head and neck.

- Each segment connects and supports the next. If you squat and the segments are not aligned, compression in unwanted areas occurs with potentially damaging effects.

Advanced squat exercises require more core strength. If you are doing a hard lower-body training day, don't start with abdominal or low-back exercises, as you'll need their full power and cooperation for proper squats.

It warrants a training session to learn how to perform a proper deep squat. Since the bullet points below may not cover the nuances, here's a recap: Start with a stable stance, typically shoulder-width apart. Your feet and knees will be in alignment and must remain in the same direction during the entire movement. With your upper body stable, meaning up-right and neutral, bend the knees and squat until your thighs are parallel to the floor. Keep your weight back on your heels and your knees behind your toes. Coming up, lead vertically from your eyes and head so that you don't bend forward.

Common mistakes when doing squats include improper knee alignment, exaggerating the back arch when lifting, and sticking the buttocks too far behind you. This shifts the balance of the weight off your legs and into your lower spine, back, and knees. Unhealthy compression of the spine and soft tissue increases the risk of injury.

Correct Squat Position Start

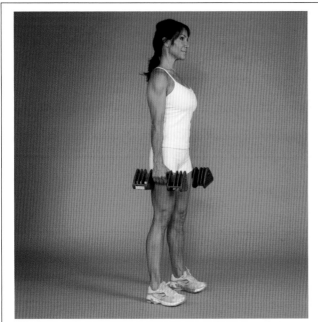

- Stand with neutral body position, feet shoulder-width apart, and shoulders retracted.

- Engage your abdominals and stablize your core.

- Toes and knees should be facing forward and aligned.

Correct Squat Position Finish

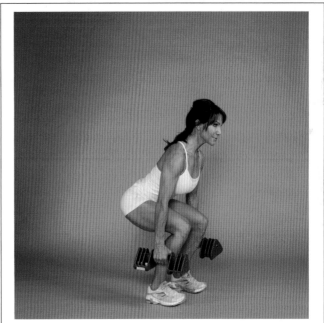

- Maintain neutral spine with a natural curve. Keep knees behind the toes and in alignment with the upper leg and feet.

- Center weight between the balls of feet and heels. Hold dumbbells vertically, following gravity.

- Contract your abdominals, supporting your spine.

PLIÉ SQUAT

For toning and shaping your thighs and buttocks, the award goes to the plié squat

The plié squat, also called the sumo squat, uses a position in which your feet are roughly twice shoulder-width apart and your toes are pointed outward. Dancers call this a *turn out*, and a squat in this position engages different muscles than a regular squat. The muscles activated during a plié squat are the gluteus maximus, the quads, hamstrings, and adductors, or inner thighs. Let's spend a moment on your gluteus maximus muscle. It deserves greater attention, as it is the largest and most superficial of the three gluteal muscles. It is what shapes your buttocks. Your buttocks allow you to sit upright without needing to rest your weight on your hands and feet like four-legged animals do. (See, it does have a purpose!)

Plié Squat: Position 1

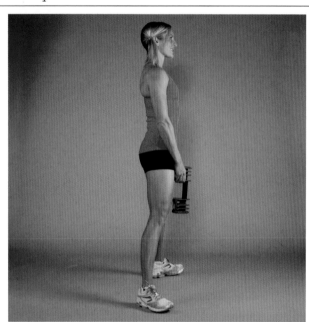

- Place your feet in an extra-wide stance. Assume neutral body position.

- Point toes out at a comfortable angle, knees aligned with toes.

- Hold the top of the dumbbell with both hands between your legs.

- Retract your shoulders and engage your abdominals.

Plié Squat: Position 2

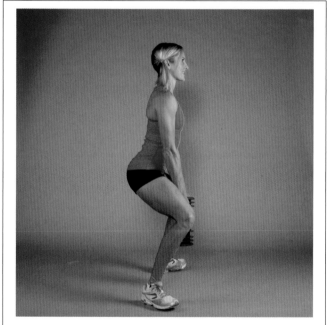

- Maintain neutral spine.

- Lower into squat by bending your knees. Knees should track over your toes.

- Keep weight on your heels.

Women tend to have wider and thicker buttocks than men because of higher subcutaneous fat and wider hips. Subcutaneous fat is found just beneath the skin and will decrease with diet and exercise. The key to losing fat on your backside demands discipline and persistence.

Plié squats have been shown to be one of the most effective exercises to shape and tone the buttocks and thighs. Add an upper-body combination exercise and you'll increase your heart rate and burn more calories.

Plié Squat: Position 3

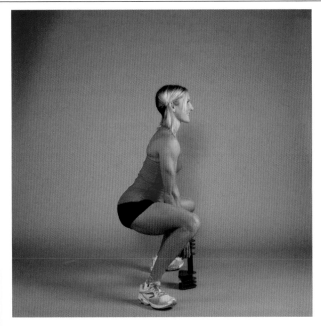

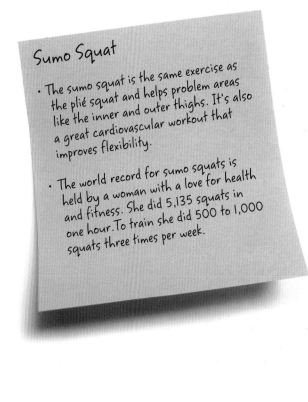

Sumo Squat

- The sumo squat is the same exercise as the plié squat and helps problem areas like the inner and outer thighs. It's also a great cardiovascular workout that improves flexibility.

- The world record for sumo squats is held by a woman with a love for health and fitness. She did 5,135 squats in one hour. To train she did 500 to 1,000 squats three times per week.

- Continue lowering your body by bending your knees until thighs are parallel to the floor.

- Keep your upper body erect and pelvis tucked while body weight remains toward heels.

- Arms and dumbbell will drop in a vertical line toward the floor.

OVERHEAD RESISTANCE SQUAT
The deep overhead squat helps determine if you need more mobility or stability work

Overhead resistance is the most challenging of all squat exercises. It also provides an immediate assessment of any weakness you may have in your musculoskeletal system. The musculoskeletal system, also known as the locomotor system, is what gives us the ability to move using our muscles and skeleton.

The body has 206 bones that meet at joints. Most of the joints are free moving, making the human skeleton flexible and mobile. If the interconnected parts of the body necessary for doing a squat exercise are immobile or unstable, it manifests itself in pronounced ways.

Check your progress with a deep, overhead squat: Can you

Resistance Squat Start

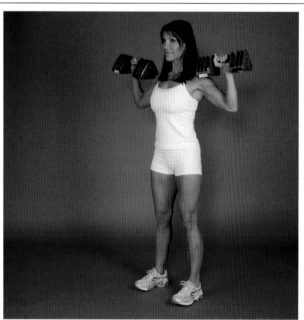

Resistance Squat Finish

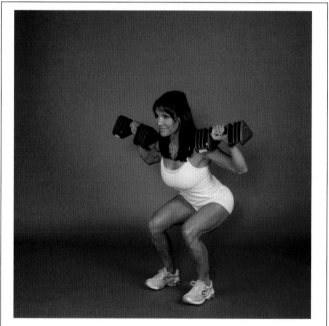

- Stand with feet shoulder-width apart and in neutral body position.

- Hold dumbbells above your shoulders with palms forward.

- In correct alignment, you will feel the weight of the dumbbells distributed down through your body into the floor.

- Weight is balanced.

- Maintain neutral spine while lowering your body by bending your knees until thighs are parallel to the floor.

- Keep your torso as upright as possible, with weight to-

ward the heels. This is more challenging with dumbbells above your shoulders than at the sides.

- Variation: Press weights over head. Use a barbell.

keep your upper back upright during a deep squat with both arms high overhead? Is your upper torso parallel to your shins? Are your thighs below horizontal with your knees aligned over your feet? Can you do this keeping both toes pointing forward, without letting your knees turn out? Lastly, are your hands still overhead so that if you dropped a vertical reference line down, it would align over your feet?

Assess your progress during a squat to find out what it means if you can't do it. If your heel comes off the floor, you have calf and ankle inflexibility. If your toes turn out, you

have weak or tight lateral calf muscles or hamstrings, or you may have weak inner thighs. If your knees drift inward, you have weak glutes and tight inner thighs. If you're not able to keep your feet straight ahead and/or you can't keep them flat and/or your thighs won't go below horizontal, you have joint restriction. If your back folds forward, you have tight hip flexors, a weak core, and poor posture. If your arms can't go overhead, your upper back lacks mobility and your shoulders are unstable.

One-Arm Overhead Squat Start

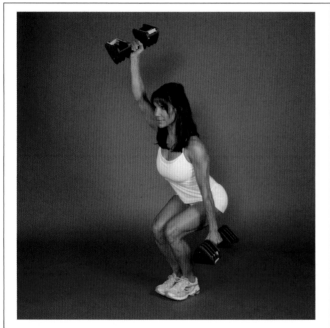

- Stand with feet and legs together in neutral body position.

- Retract shoulders and engage abdominals.

- Lower your body by bending the knees until thighs are almost parallel to the floor.

- Hold dumbbells so palms are facing each other. Raise right arm overhead.

One-Arm Overhead Squat Finish

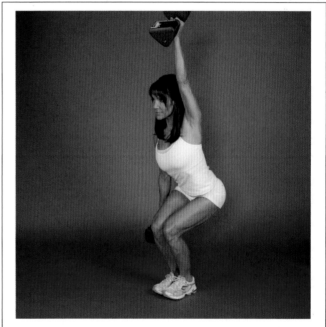

- Return to standing position while maintaining neutral spine.

- Simultaneously lower your right arm to the side, keeping dumbbell close to your body.

- Repeat squat motion and raise left arm overhead.

- Choose a weight based on your shoulder strength, not your leg strength.

CLEAN AND PRESS

The clean and press is a compound exercise, engaging most of the muscles used in daily lifting

The clean and press is a highly functional exercise that will get you in shape. You use some or all of these movements daily, from lifting an item off the floor to placing one in an overhead cupboard. If this were the only big strength exercise you did daily, odds are you'd see results.

This exercise is ideal if you have a busy schedule and are trying to keep fit with a minimal investment of training and time. It also has the benefit of increasing your functional capacity for daily tasks.

The American College of Sports Medicine found the press phase of the exercise to be the most difficult task for people over age 70. This unfortunate reality can be addressed with

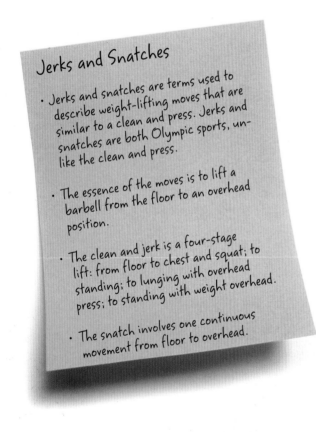

Jerks and Snatches

- Jerks and snatches are terms used to describe weight-lifting moves that are similar to a clean and press. Jerks and snatches are both Olympic sports, unlike the clean and press.

- The essence of the moves is to lift a barbell from the floor to an overhead position.

- The clean and jerk is a four-stage lift: from floor to chest and squat; to standing; to lunging with overhead press; to standing with weight overhead.

- The snatch involves one continuous movement from floor to overhead.

Clean and Press: Position 1

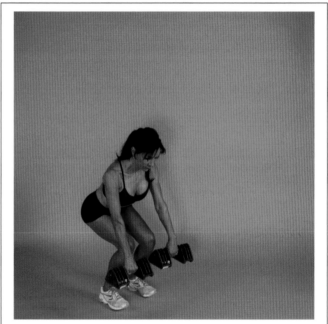

- Stand with feet shoulder-width apart, toes forward, and neutral body position.

- With weights on the floor in front of your feet, squat down and grab the dumbbells with palms facing back.

- Retract your shoulders and engage your abdominals.

- Begin to stand by contracting your glutes and quads. Keep your arms straight.

strength training and maintaining functional fitness.

Maintaining functionality throughout life, referred to as *compression of morbidity*, is a practical way to extend the useful years of life. Morbidity is a disease or condition that impairs bodily functions. Most people in the United States reach morbidity decades before mortality. To avoid having your retirement years equate to a rapid decline in health, stay strong and active. Think "An ounce of prevention is worth a pound of cure." Don't wait until you have a physical problem to start training.

Clean and Press: Position 2

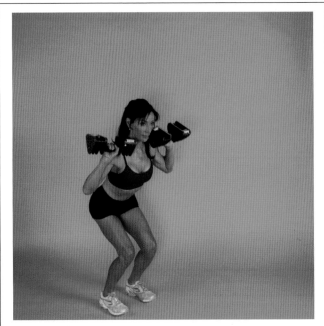

- Firmly grip the dumbbells.

- Continue the upward movement. Bend elbows and flip your wrists to position the dumbbells at your shoulders in one continuous motion.

- The dumbbells are now resting in your palms with wrists flexed.

Clean and Press: Position 3

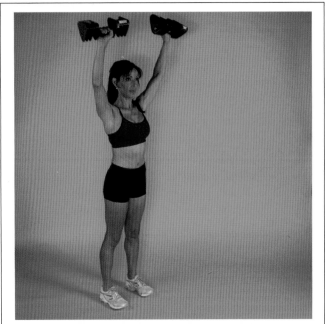

- Press through the heels and come to a standing position while raising the dumbbells overhead.

- Throughout the movement body weight remains toward the heels, knees stay

behind toes, and back does not round.

- Keep shoulders retracted when weights are overhead.

- Reverse the movement to return dumbbells to the floor.

STABILITY SQUAT

Squatting on an uneven surface improves your balance and adds a new challenge to training

Wobble boards and inflatable discs are part of the functional fitness arsenal for rehabilitation, developing balance, increasing confidence, stimulating reflexes, and improving performance, agility, range of motion, strength, and coordination. Wobble boards are excellent ankle strengtheners and help prevent injuries.

The wobble board is about 16 inches in diameter and has a nonslip surface on top and a single, small ball, or rail, on the bottom. This requires one to balance on the platform to keep an even stance. The rocker version, a variation of the wobble board shown here, has a larger surface area and provides more stability.

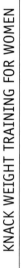

Wobble Board Squat Start

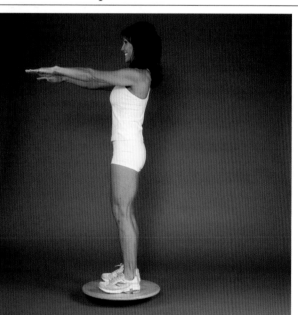

- Stand with feet hip-width apart, centered on the wobble board.

- Maintain neutral body position. Raise arms to front at shoulder height.

- Concentrate on actively using inner thighs and upper hips to balance.

- Do not let knees bow out to the sides or cave in to center.

Wobble Board Squat Finish

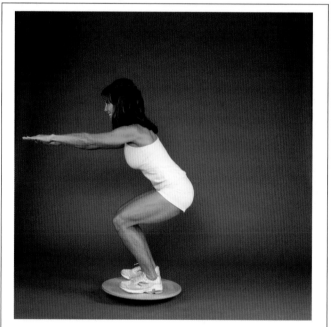

- After balancing, bend knees, lowering into a quarter-squat.

- Focus on aligning hips, knees, and ankles. Keep knees behind toes.

- Hold the squat position for a moment before returning to standing.

- You may find it easier to balance in a squat position than standing.

Practice exercises that will improve your balance and strength before you perform a full squat exercise on this unstable surface. Balancing on two feet without the edges of the board touching the floor helps get you comfortable. Once mastered, rock forward, backward, and to the sides to activate the muscles in the ankles. The one-foot balance is next. Continue into a two-legged squat and eventually a one-legged squat.

You may find that squatting is actually easier than standing. Your center of gravity is lower when you squat, which helps you balance. Make sure that you still maintain all rules for good form and neutral body position while on a wobble board.

Soon you will be able to incorporate the wobble board into your functional-training program and will use it to perform push-ups, lunges, and weight-training exercises. Adding variety to your program keeps you interested and helps longevity and consistency with training.

Stability Disc Squat Start

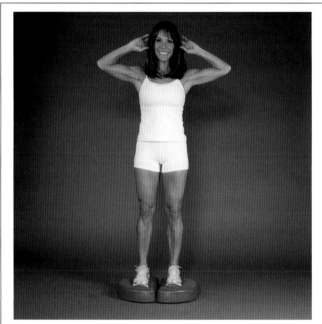

- Pillow-style stability discs come in many shapes and sizes. They are pre-filled with air.

- Stand on disc, feet hip-width apart.

- Maintain neutral body position. Place hands behind head, elbows out to sides.

- Concentrate on actively using inner thighs and upper hips to maintain alignment.

Stability Disc Squat Finish

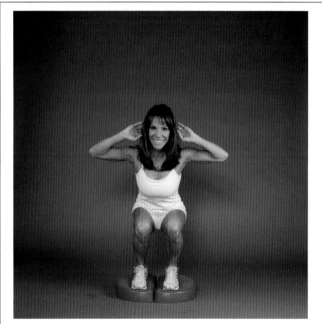

- This should feel easier than squatting on a wobble board.

- Bend knees and lower into a full squat until your thighs are parallel to the floor.

- Keep your knees behind your toes and aligned with your upper legs and feet.

- Straighten your legs to return to standing position.

ONE-LEG SQUAT

Squatting will impressively improve the look, muscularity, and strength of the abdominal muscles

Stabilizing contractions build muscle. If you are performing squats regularly, your abdominals, which stabilize your body during a squat, will get stronger, along with your gluteus, hamstrings, quadriceps, and back. That doesn't mean you should stop lower abdominal training, but it is an indication of how important squats are for your total body physique.

One-leg squats are considered one of the most effective sport-specific resistance conditioning exercises available. Training the legs independently permits the development of symmetrical leg strength. Your core muscles, in addition to keeping you firmly stable in the up-down movement, will help you from falling over to the side. Lateral stability and balance relies on

One-Leg Squat: Position 1

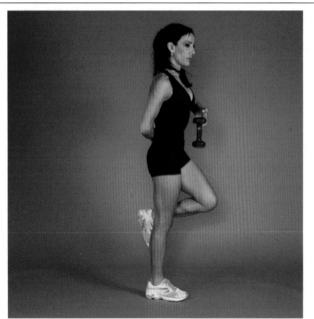

- Stand in neutral body position, holding the top of the dumbbell in your left hand.

- Bring left foot to right knee, balancing on one leg. Place your right arm behind your back at a 90-degree angle.

One-Leg Squat: Position 2

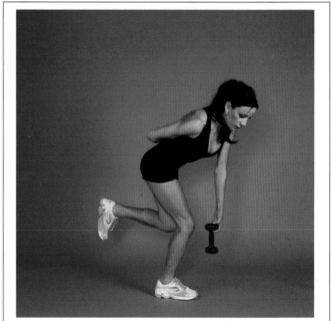

- Retract shoulders and engage abdominals.

- Begin squatting with your right leg while bending forward with the dumbbell at vertical.

- Your left foot will cross behind your right leg for balance.

- Maintain neutral spine and head alignment.

your obliques, or side abdominals, and lower back muscles.

To aid balance, *dab* with your foot during the squat. Essentially, you place the unsupported foot lightly on the floor to keep you from toppling. The key to all balance moves is to look up and straight ahead.

When performing most balance moves, stop the exercise when your form starts to suffer. The physical challenge of balance causes fatigue mentally and physically. It is demanding to the nervous system. This explains why some days, when you're tired, you just don't have your normal coordination.

One-Leg Squat: Position 3

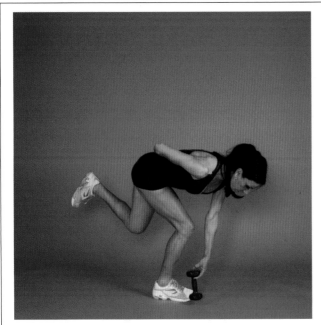

- Squat lower and bend forward to tap dumbbell on the floor.

- Your left foot will rise slightly. Keep your right knee behind your toe even when bending forward.

- Press through your heels to return to standing position by extending your right leg using buttocks and thigh muscles.

- Repeat on other side.

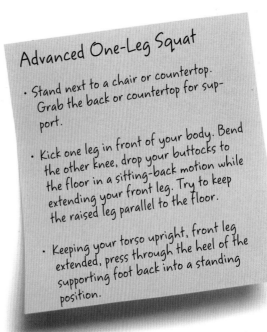

Advanced One-Leg Squat

- Stand next to a chair or countertop. Grab the back or countertop for support.

- Kick one leg in front of your body. Bend the other knee, drop your buttocks to the floor in a sitting-back motion while extending your front leg. Try to keep the raised leg parallel to the floor.

- Keeping your torso upright, front leg extended, press through the heel of the supporting foot back into a standing position.

WALL SQUAT

Adding a stability ball to the wall squat turns the exercise from an isometric to a compound movement

Wall squats target the gluteus muscles, abdomen, back, and thighs. They can be performed anywhere wall space is available. Not only will your posture improve from doing wall squats, your lower-body strength will improve. Without a stability ball, a wall squat with your body weight in a static position is an example of an isometric exercise.

During an isometric contraction, the muscle exerts an equal amount of force as the amount of resistance. This means there is muscle contraction with no movement. During periods of sitting or standing, your body is engaged in isometric exercise. The more postural strength you have, the less your muscles will fatigue.

Wall Squat: Position 1

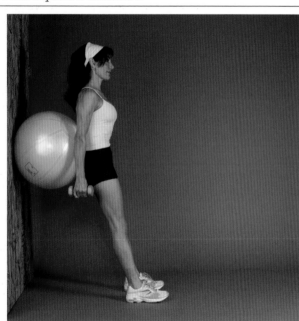

- Grab dumbbells with your palms facing each other.

- Place ball against the wall and lean into it with the small of your back.

- Position feet in front of your body with dumbbells at your sides.

- Maintain neutral body position.

- Retract your shoulders and engage your abdominals.

Wall Squat: Position 2

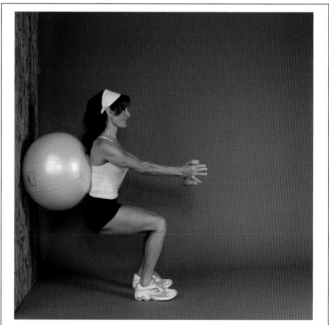

- Squat and roll the ball with your back until your legs form a 90-degree angle. Keep weight toward the heels.

- Lengthen spine, retract shoulders, and engage abdominals to prevent bouncing against the ball.

- Perform front raise palms facing each other.

- Variation: lateral raise.

Isometrics can increase strength, but there are disadvantages. Isometrics increase blood pressure more than conventional strength-training exercise. You don't put your muscles through a full range of motion, and you don't get the stretching benefits. Stretching is the stimulus that helps muscles grow. After time, lack of stretching will cause you to lose flexibility.

Use a stability ball to make your wall-squat a full compound strength-training exercise (not an isometric hold). You'll love the improved flexibility, strength, cardiorespiratory endurance, agility, and balance gains.

Wall Squat: Position 3

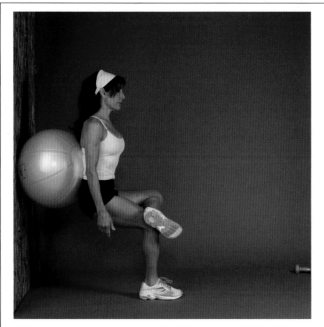

- Ditch the dumbbells.

- Maintain squat position, keeping arms by your sides.

- Place left foot over right knee and balance in a one-leg wall squat.

- Try to hold the squat for a minimum of ten seconds.

- Variation: Cross left leg over your right knee while standing, and then lower into squat position.

Wall Squat: Position 4

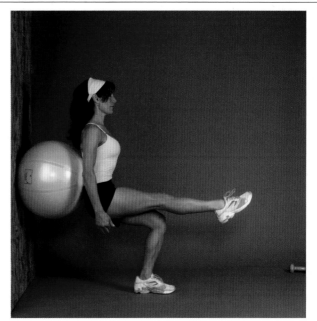

- Return your left foot to the floor.

- Extend right leg straight in front of your body, parallel to the floor, and balance in a one-leg squat. Hold for a minimum of ten seconds.

- Repeat other side.

- Variation: Raise right leg while standing and lower into squat position.

133

STATIC LUNGE

Change lunge progression in small increments to avoid pain, injury, and frustration

In a static exercise, the feet do not move; the body travels up and down during the exercise. The static lunge is also called the static split squat. Using body weight alone, or adding dumbbells for resistance, this a great exercise for beginners and avanced level training.

As with all lunge exercises, you feel the effort in all the ma-

jor muscles of the hips, buttocks, and thighs. When asked if she was sore from doing lunges, one woman summed it up well by saying, "Who lowered the toilet?" Sitting or squatting can be painful when you have delayed-onset muscle soreness from challenging workouts.

Let's review delayed-onset muscle soreness. It typically oc-

Static Lunge Start

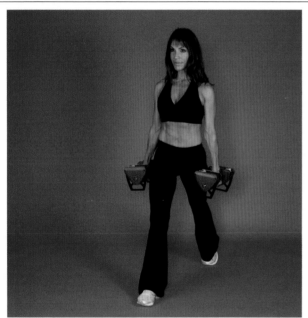

- Stand with right foot forward, left foot back. Distance between feet should be approximately the length of your leg.

- Grab dumbbells, palms facing each other by your sides.

- Keep weight evenly distributed between your legs; hold hips square, upper body erect, and shoulders retracted.

Static Lunge Finish

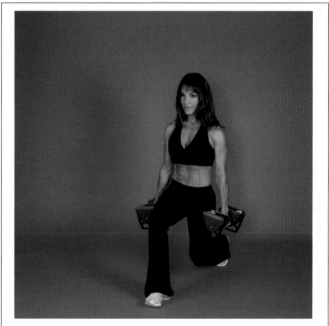

- Bend your legs, dropping your left knee straight toward the floor and keeping your right knee behind the toes.

- Weight remains evenly distributed. Do not twist or lift one hip higher.

- Return to standing by pressing your weight into your heel, contracting the quads, glutes, and hamstrings.

- Repeat with other leg.

curs after eccentric or negative movements, such as running downhill or lowering your body weight. The cause of pain is still unknown, although there is no question it exists. The soreness is thought to be a result of muscle cell damage or microtears in the muscle fibers. If you experience stiffness, swelling, strength loss, and pain after exercising, give yourself two to three days to recover.

Mild stretching may help speed recovery from soreness. Don't overstretch, because this can aggravate the condition. Alternating cold and warm showers helps increase circula-

tion. Massage therapy is also helpful.

As your fitness increases, you can make the static lunge more challenging by progressing from both feet on the floor to placing one foot on a step or bench. This also increases your range of motion during the exercise. Make sure that your fitness and flexibility are sufficient to support your body in this exposed position, especially if using dumbbells.

Front Leg Elevated Static Lunge

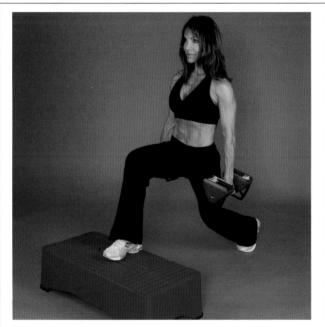

- Placing front foot on a platform increases range of motion and provides additional quad and hip-flexor stretch.

- Position front foot on a sturdy step and back foot on the floor.

- Grab dumbbells with palms facing each other by your sides. Use same movement as static lunge.

- The challenge is to keep your hips square.

Back Leg Elevated Static Lunge

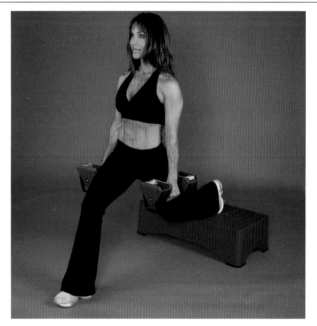

- Place ball of back foot on a sturdy step and front foot on the floor.

- Take time to position your front foot, as this move requires a lot of balance. Take

caution that the knee is not overstressed.

- Grab dumbbells with palms facing each other by your sides. Use same movement as static lunge.

REVERSE LUNGE

Trainers rarely have clients perform a front lunge due to the strain on the knee

Front lunges have the stigma of being harmful to the knee. And when performed incorrectly, they are. However, a properly executed front lunge is safe for the joints and an extremely beneficial exercise. Front lunges are an effective way to improve tone and shape to the buttocks, hips, and thighs. To ensure proper execution requires a mirror and astute at-

tention or the guidance of a certified personal trainer.

Alternatively, you can do a reverse lunge, which provides the same muscular benefits as the front lunge but is easier to perform correctly. The reverse lunge uses the same ultimate position as a front lunge, but instead of stepping forward, you step backward. This difference helps prevent the ten-

Reverse Lunge: Position 1

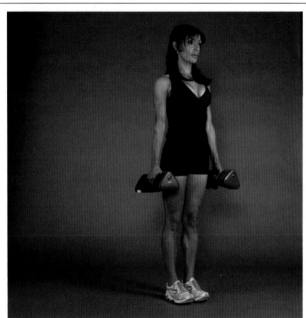

- Stand with neutral body position. Grab dumbbells with palms facing each other.

- When preparing to lunge backward with your right leg, subtly shift your body weight to your left foot without moving away from the center line.

- Retract your shoulders and engage your abdominals.

Reverse Lunge: Position 2

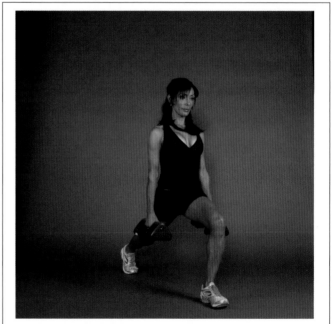

- With torso erect, extend your right leg back in a lunge while keeping your left knee behind the toes.

- Once in a lunge, distribute your weight evenly between both legs. Your left thigh is almost parallel to the floor and your right leg extended. Knee should not touch floor.

dency to lean too far into the front knee, causing it to extend over the toes.

When doing any type of lunge, it is key to remember to weight both feet evenly. You may naturally want to focus on and place more weight on your front leg, because it may feel more stable. However, greater stability and safety for your knees requires equal work by both legs. One easy way to remember this is to simply focus on weighting your back leg.

Reverse Lunge: Position 3

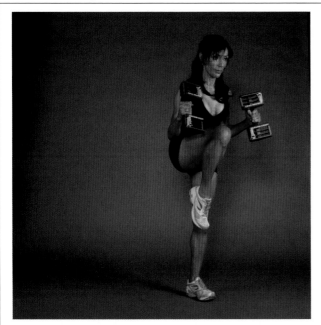

- Return to upright position by pressing weight into your left heel, contracting the muscles in your legs, glutes, and hips.

- Without touching your right foot to the floor, continue lifting your right knee to the chest. Contract your abdominals while performing a hammer biceps curl.

- Return to standing.

- Repeat with other leg.

Standing Leg Raise

- Build up your standing knee crunch endurance by practicing a standing leg raise.

- Keep your back straight and your arms by your sides. Smoothly raise one knee until your thigh is parallel to the floor while activating your transversus abdominus. Hold this position for five to ten seconds while keeping your hips square.

- Return to start position and repeat on the same side to build endurance. Then, after finishing your set (six holds), switch sides.

SIDE, ANTI-ROTATION LUNGE

Practice side lunges after you have built a fitness base with static and reverse lunges

Side lunges cover the spectrum of thigh-muscle training. The movement involves bending one knee while stretching the opposite leg to the side. It is a dynamic, athletic movement recommended for advanced fitness levels. In addition to working the quads, hamstrings, and glutes, side lunges also engage the inner and outer thighs (adductors and abductors).

Make sure to work up to a side lunge by starting off with static lunges. You can then progress to an elevated static lunge, both forward and back off the platform, and then to a reverse lunge. If your training has thus far been focused on stable surfaces, consider placing a wobble board or stability disc under foot during the static and reverse lunge exercises.

Side Lunge Start

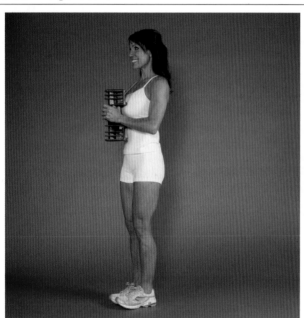

- Stand in neutral body position, legs and feet together with one dumbbell held close to the body at chest level.

- Retract your shoulders and engage your abdominals.

- Feet remain pointed straight out in front of your body throughout the movement.

Side Lunge Finish

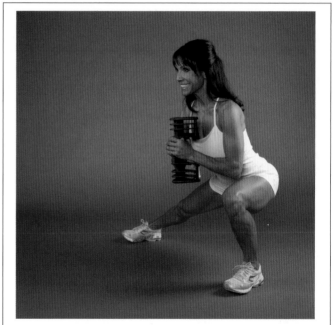

- Step out to the left side, keeping your right foot stationary. Your right leg will be in full extension. Do not lock your knee.

- Keep upper body upright and left knee aligned over your foot, behind toes.

- Focus on front and inner thigh muscles to return to standing. Repeat on other leg.

Using resistance may not be necessary if you have not exhausted your capabilities for body-weight-only balance and stability training. Additional resistance is only necessary when your body has reached a point of proficiency. If the workout is easy, you need to add challenge. This enables your muscles to continue to get stronger. Again, progress little by little and make sure you are performing exercises with a full range of motion and proper form.

Another lunge variation is the anti-rotation lunge. This increases your balance and precision simultaneously. You will need an elastic toner for this exercise. The toner, anchored to a door or solid surface at about chest level, acts as your resistance. When standing perpendicular to the outstretched band and holding it taut in front of you, you need to use your core strength to maintain centered balance.

Engaging your abdominals and keeping an erect upper body during lunges are crucial. Holding your head high and retracting your shoulders will help keep you from rotating or swaying.

Anti-Rotation Lunge Start

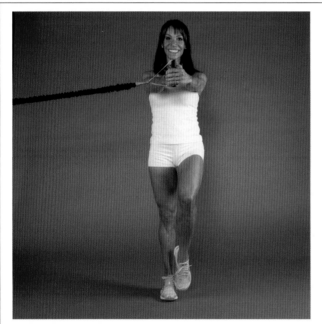

- Anchor toner at chest level. Stand with your right side to anchor and grab the handle with palms together.

- Balance on your right leg and lift your left foot slightly off the floor. Place toe or heel against the other leg for balance.

- Extend arms to front, keeping toner tight.

Anti-Rotation Lunge Finish

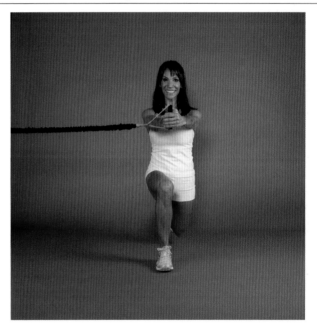

- With shoulders retracted and abdominals engaged, lunge your left leg back until your right thigh is parallel to the floor.

- Keep tension in the toner throughout the movement.

- This creates the lateral balance challenge.

- Step back to start. Repeat on other side.

- Variation: Place stability disc under front foot.

WALKING LUNGE

Next time you walk down the hall, drop down and sneak in a few lunges

Changing your step from an upright casual stride to a walking lunge will improve your fitness while still getting you where you need to go! All the benefits of lunges discussed previously also apply to walking lunges. In addition, you gain flexibility in your hip flexors. Because of the constant movement, your heart rate increases, making walking lunges a

conditioning exercise for your aerobic system. Even if you are in great shape, walking lunges are a workout. Ten paces can be challenging when done mindfully.

Walking lunges are compromising to the knee if you do not keep your form in check. To keep your knee out of harm's way, apply the same neutral body position and alignment

Walking Lunge: Position 1

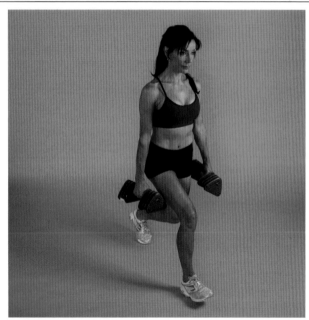

- Use light dumbbells, hold with palms facing each other.

- Step forward with right foot.

- Keep hips square and front knee behind toes as you bend your knees, lowering into a lunge position.

- Keep head neutral or look up.

Walking Lunge: Position 2

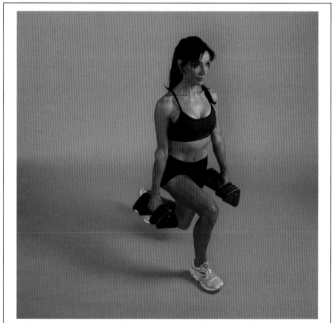

- Keep hips square and front knee behind toes as you bend your knees more, lowering your body deeper into a lunge.

- Only lunge as low as is comfortable.

- Press your weight into your right heel to return to upright position.

- During pass through, left foot will not rest on the floor.

we covered in previous chapters: Keep an upright torso and don't lean forward; use your back leg for stability; do not let your front knee go beyond your toe; and make sure your front foot is weighted evenly, through the heel.

Momentum should not be employed during a walking lunge. With each step forward, pause at the top before your next stride out. Intensity can be added by holding dumbbells.

If you are looking for another unique approach to spice up the walking lunge, try exponential lunges by adding multiple reps or static lunges to each step.

Walking Lunge: Position 3

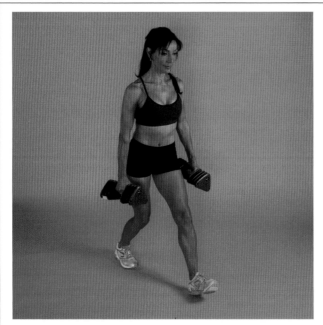

- Keep your upper torso erect, shoulders retracted, and abdominals engaged during transition to next step.

- Bring your left leg back in front of your body, landing softly on your foot. Concentrate on back leg strength for stability, keeping hips square to the floor.

- Dumbbells remain by your sides.

Walking Lunge: Position 4

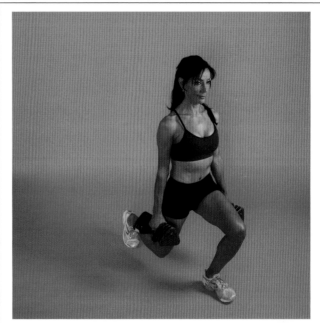

- Continue walking lunge sequence one step at a time.

- Modification: No weights.

- Variation: Exponential lunge technique—perform multiple static lunges in between each step.

141

BIG STEP-UP
Women gain the majority of their weight in the hips, buttocks, and thighs

It makes sense that women would want to train their backside. The hips, buttocks, and thighs are where ladies tend to carry extra body fat. Since spot reducing does not exist, exercise must happen. If you are looking to burn calories and tone your body, you must build lean muscle. The more lean muscle mass, the more fat burning you will experience—

during and after your workout.

The step-up is an excellent strength-training exercise that will strengthen the large muscles in your lower body. It will also prepare you for real-life climbing. Mountain climbers have used stair-step machines and step-up exercises to train for expeditions. Even if you are not climbing a mountain in

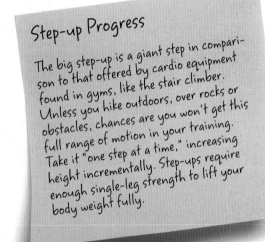

Step-up Progress

The big step-up is a giant step in comparison to that offered by cardio equipment found in gyms, like the stair climber. Unless you hike outdoors, over rocks or obstacles, chances are you won't get this full range of motion in your training. Take it "one step at a time," increasing height incrementally. Step-ups require enough single-leg strength to lift your body weight fully.

Big Step-up: Position 1

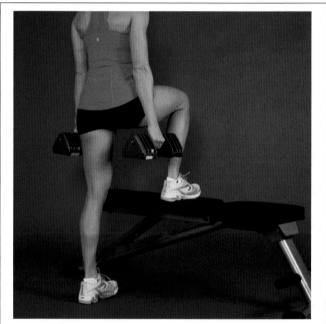

- Stand behind a bench or 15-inch platform, dumbbells in hand, palms facing each other.

- Retract your shoulders and engage your abdominals.

- Place right foot on the bench and transfer your weight to your left heel.

- Hips should be square to the floor.

the near future, you will benefit from being able to skip the elevator without working up a sweat.

Stair-step machines (not shown), found in most gyms, mimic walking up stairs. They resemble an escalator, only you have to move your legs. You can continue as long as your legs and cardio fitness endures. Most machines allow a range of step sizes, depending on how high you lift your knee. Make sure not to cheat by taking ministeps. Step-ups onto a fixed object prevent cheating, as you must pick up your leg the same height every time to complete the repetition.

MAKE IT EASY

You need strong knee stability and quadriceps muscles to control the eccentric movement of a step-down. When coming off the step, the bent knee causes the quad muscle to lengthen (an eccentric contraction). Eccentric movements recruit more fast-twitch muscle fibers. Don't let gravity pull you down; step down deliberately, slowly, and gently to maximize muscular strength benefits.

Big Step-up: Position 2

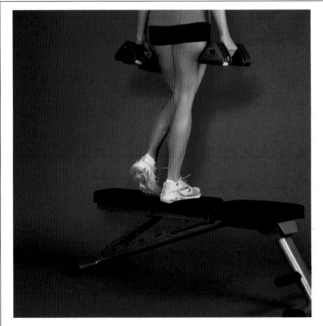

- With upper body erect, push weight into your right heel, lifting your body onto the bench.

- Concentrate on using only your right leg; use your left leg for balance. Tap your left toe on the bench at top.

- Avoid leaning your upper body forward or lifting one hip higher than the other when stepping up.

Big Step-up: Position 3

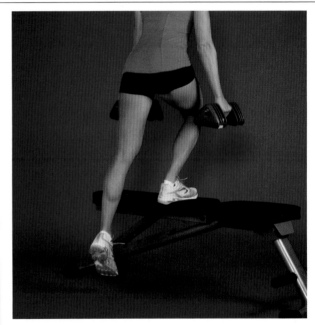

- With an erect upper body, slowly step back down with your left foot, keeping weight on your right heel.

- Control the movement so your left foot lands gently.

- Allow your right foot to follow until standing on the floor with both feet.

- Repeat with left step-up, right step-down.

STABILITY FLEX LUNGE
Mind-body exercise is a physical exercise executed with a profound inwardly directed focus

Any time you combine exercises, you get more total-body training benefits. In addition to working the leg and buttocks muscles as any lunge does, the stability flex lunge incorporates stretching and crunching of the abdominal muscles. You will not need any dumbbells or added resistance for this exercise.

The stability flex lunge is more movement and posture based than dynamic and fast-paced. Being methodical with your exercise can transform your body. This means striving for perfect movements, perfect body alignment, and perfect frame of mind. Focus on the moment.

Every lunge brings you a step closer to slim hips, long lean

Flex Lunge: Position 1

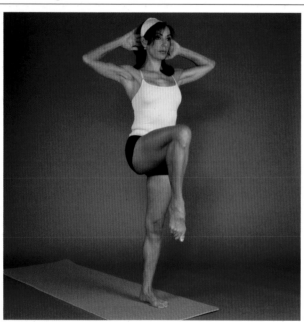

- Start with hips square.

- Stand in neutral body position at the top of a mat with hands behind your head, elbows out to the sides of your body.

- Retract your shoulders and engage your abdominals.

- Lift your right knee until your thigh is parallel to the floor, balancing on your left leg.

Flex Lunge: Position 2

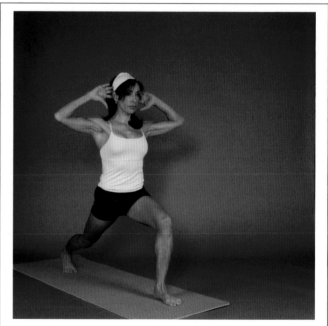

- Maintain upper-body position and lunge back with your right leg.

- Keep your hips square and weight balanced between legs.

- Keep your left knee behind toes with feet, lower legs, and upper legs in alignment.

muscles, and a high tight derrière. Losing weight will show off your assets once your body fat levels have decreased. Remember: Changes in body composition, the ratio of body fat to lean body mass, are not reflected in the number on the scale. Have your body fat tested by a professional every six to eight weeks if you are on a weight-loss program.

Personal trainers and fitness centers provide this service. The Accu-Measure body fat caliper and the Tanita bioelectric impedance analysis scale are consumer friendly for home testing if that's your preference.

ZOOM

If you are on an extreme diet and have just begun a weight-lifting routine, do not rely on the bathroom scale to measure success. Fad diets will most likely cause you to lose both body fat and lean muscle tissue. Because muscle is denser than body fat, you should gauge your resistance training progress on how your clothes fit before looking at the scale.

Flex Lunge: Position 3

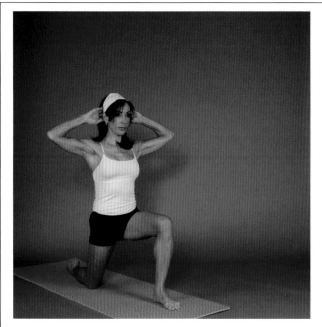

- Keep upper-body position the same.

- Gently lower your right knee to the mat, keeping weight off the kneecap.

- Balance your weight between lower right leg and top of foot and left heel and quad.

- Pressing weight into left heel and engaging your abdominals will help to stabilize.

Flex Lunge: Position 4

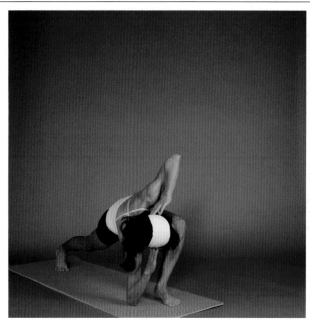

- Lift your right knee off the mat and return to lunge position with leg extended.

- Keeping hands behind your head and elbows out to the sides, rotate your torso and tap your right elbow to the mat.

- Keep your body lengthened and centered.

- Repeat with other side.

LEG-UP LIFT

Seek to have a balanced ratio of strength between your hamstrings and quadriceps

Technically, the hamstring is one of the tendons behind the knee. There are three muscles that make up the back side of the upper leg: the semitendinosus, the semimenbranosus, and the biceps femoris. The word *ham* originally referred to the fat and muscle behind the knee. The word *string* described the tendons. Together, *hamstring* became common

vernacular when referring to the upper, back of the leg.

The hamstrings bend or flex the knees and straighten or extend the hips. They play a critical role in daily activities, like walking, running, and squatting. Weak hamstrings are prone to injury. A pulled or strained hamstring is an excessive stretch or tear of muscle fibers and related tissue. It is a

Leg-up Lift Start

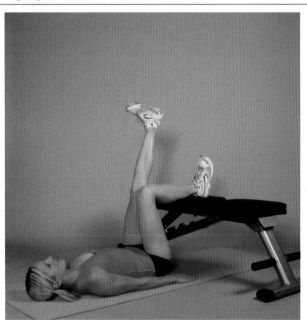

- Lying on the floor, place your right heel on a bench. Flex the foot so toes point toward the ceiling.

- Extend your left leg straight up, flexing the foot.

- Keep head and spine aligned and hips square. Place your arms at your sides, palms flat on the floor.

Leg-up Lift Finish

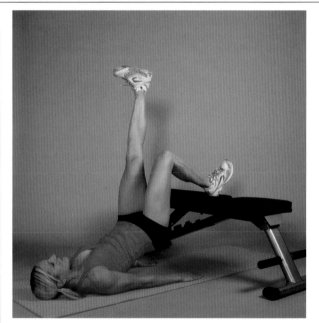

- Keep your head, upper back, and palms on the floor while pressing the right heel into the bench. Contract hamstrings to lift buttocks. Keep your left leg straight.

- If upper body slides away from bench, you are pressing your right foot away instead of straight down.

- Repeat with other leg.

146

common injury in sports and can be prevented with weight training.

Hamstring inflexibility is a rampant problem; more stretching and forward bending is needed. If you have chronic tightness in your hamstrings, focus on hamstring exercises that increase flexibility until you develop more range of motion.

It is imperative that you maintain muscular balance on the front and back side of your legs. A thorough leg workout should include exercises for both quads and hamstrings.

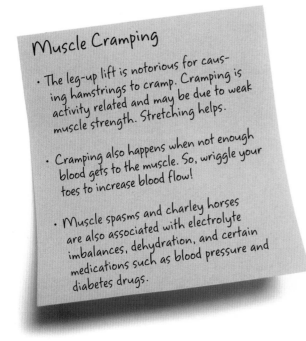

Muscle Cramping

- The leg-up lift is notorious for causing hamstrings to cramp. Cramping is activity related and may be due to weak muscle strength. Stretching helps.

- Cramping also happens when not enough blood gets to the muscle. So, wriggle your toes to increase blood flow!

- Muscle spasms and charley horses are also associated with electrolyte imbalances, dehydration, and certain medications such as blood pressure and diabetes drugs.

ZOOM

The leg-up lift is a made-up name. Many trainers come up with names that describe a movement. This exercise is one of the few hamstring workout options that you can do without machines or special equipment. Incorporate the leg-up lift as a supplement to your hamstring training and use it when traveling.

Stability Leg-up Lift

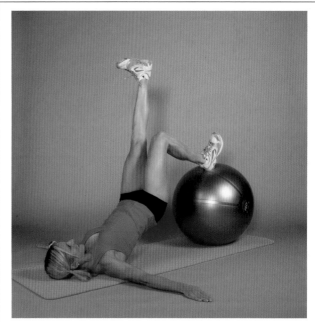

- Use same body position as the bench exercise; place heel on top of the ball.

- To balance during the lift, position hands out to the sides of your body and

press firmly into the floor. Engage abdominals to stabilize your core and keep hips square.

- Repeat with other leg.

STABILITY LEG CURL
Some of the best hamstring training is functional movement involving your gluteus muscles and legs

Your hamstrings get a workout every time you perform compound strength-training movements like squats, lunges, and step-ups. If you are a cyclist and use clipless pedals, or toe cages, you can develop nice hamstring strength during the lift portion of the pedal stroke. If you enjoy trail running, your hamstrings get a workout when you travel up and down the hills.

While a stability leg curl is not an everyday movement, it is a functional training method because it increases your balance, strength, and overall fitness, all of which transfers to life. When you do exercises that require engagement of your core, you teach your body to engage your core during everyday motions as well.

Stability Leg Curl Start

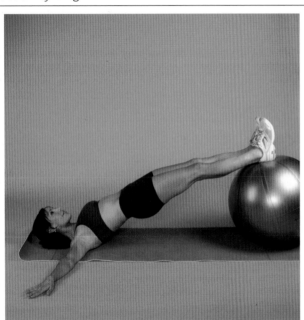

- Lie on your back with hands by your sides; place the ball under your heels.

- Rest your upper body and buttocks on the mat; stretch your arms out to your sides, palms down.

- Engage your abdominals and raise hips into a straight body bridge.

- Maintain neutral body position and keep your hips lifted.

Stability Leg Curl Finish

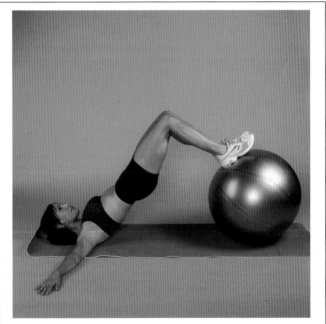

- Pull the ball to your body by curling your heels toward your buttocks.

- Keep your hips as high as possible while maintaining neutral spine.

- Push the ball back out by straightening your legs to start position.

The stability leg curl helps balance discrepancies between the quads and hamstrings. If your hamstrings are tight and your quads are weak, there is a pull on the front of the pelvis and lower back that can cause back pain and injury.

Athletes love this exercise because it dynamically strengthens the muscles around the knee joint. Use caution if you feel pain behind the knee when in the reverse plank position. It may be helpful to place the ball further up the leg, on the calf muscle to minimize the force.

············· GREEN ● LIGHT ·············

Test your hamstring and quadriceps ratio. Using a leg extension machine at the gym, see how much you can lift with your quads. Do the same with a lying leg curl machine to test your hamstrings. Your quads should be no more than one-third stronger than your hamstrings; for example, 60 and 45 pounds with your quads and hamstrings, respectively. If the difference is greater, focus more on hamstring training.

One-Leg Stability Leg Curl

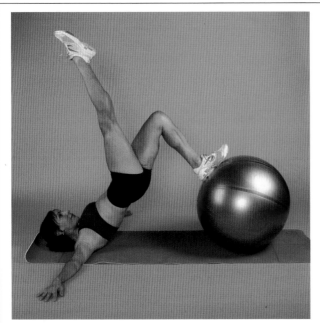

- After performing the two-leg curl, lift one foot off the ball. This is not easy!

- Keep hips lifted and maintain strict form. Avoid folding your chin into chest.

- Repeat with other leg.

- Modification: Place hands by your sides for additional challenge.

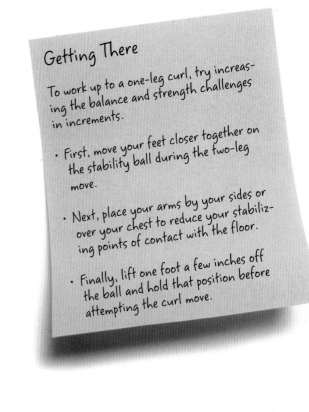

Getting There

To work up to a one-leg curl, try increasing the balance and strength challenges in increments.

- First, move your feet closer together on the stability ball during the two-leg move.

- Next, place your arms by your sides or over your chest to reduce your stabilizing points of contact with the floor.

- Finally, lift one foot a few inches off the ball and hold that position before attempting the curl move.

HAMSTRING AND CALF

149

DEAD LIFT

Considered one of the purest tests of strength, dead weight lifts date back to stone lifting

The dead lift is a compound movement that works grip strength, along with the back, abs, hamstrings, inner thighs, quads, and calves. The classic dead lift exercise uses an Olympic bar and weight plates. This form is considered the purest test of strength. Unlike other lifts, it begins on the floor, forcing you to lift "dead weight." Firefighters train extensively to

learn how to hoist passive weight. Mothers are familiar with this concept from picking up a sleeping child.

When done properly, dead lifts build back strength and help you develop good habits when lifting heavy objects from the floor. This exercise is highly functional and deserves your full attention.

Dead Lift: Position 1

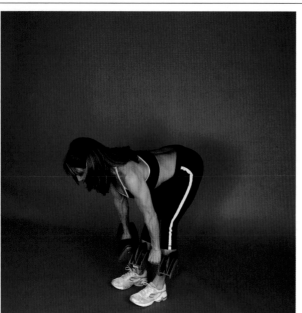

- Stand with feet hip-width apart. Squat to grab the dumbbells at your feet.

- Straighten your legs and back, maintaining neutral spine, retracted shoulders, and engaged abdominals.

- Initiate lift off the floor, using lower-body strength. Keep dumbbells close.

- Flex your legs to bring the dumbbells up to your shins.

Dead Lift: Position 2

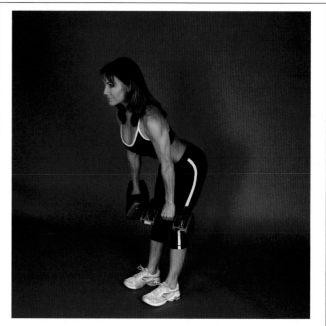

- Knees and feet point in same direction throughout the movement.

- Lift your upper body, using hip and glute strength to rise. Keep your chest up, shoulders retracted, and

abdominals engaged. Look forward.

- Push from your heels and bring hips forward. Don't pull with your lower back.

You will not injure your back doing dead lifts as long as you do them correctly. For our purposes, we won't do the exercise like the ol' stone lifters, power lifters, and Olympic competitors do. We will use dumbbells and a Romanian technique.

Dead lifts require balance and athletic coordination. They are not recommended for those with knee and back problems. Failure to maintain neutral spine during the movement can cause undue stress to the spinal discs. It is important to be proficient in the recruitment of your deep abdominal and trunk muscles.

Dead Lift: Position 3

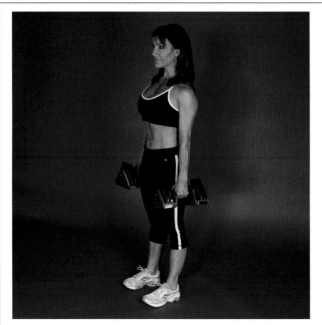

- Squeeze your glutes and inner thighs; bring hips forward to continue lifting.

- Keep weight on heels and let arms follow the pull of gravity.

- Exercise ends when knees and hips are locked but not hyperextended and body is in neutral position.

One-Leg Dead Lift

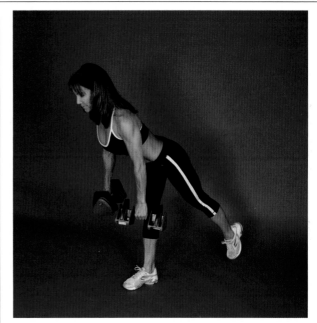

- Use same movement as the two-leg dead lift.

- Extend left leg behind your body. Concentrate on keeping your torso from rotating.

- Keep pushing from the heels. Curl toes up to force weight on the back of your foot.

- Return dumbbells below knees by flexing at hip to initiate the movement.

HAMSTRING AND CALF

LEG CURL

Female athletes experience ten times the amount of hamstring tears as men due to weakness and muscle imbalance

The leg curl exercise is an isolation movement for the hamstrings. It is a great exercise for overall development of the legs. Athletes, fitness enthusiasts, and individuals with a muscular imbalance can use the leg curl to target this area.

Fitness equipment manufacturers have machines specifically for hamstring leg curls. The options are seated, lying,

and standing one-leg versions. If you are training the hamstrings at home, you need an elastic toner to duplicate this specific leg curl move, unless you have a gym-style piece of equipment.

Executing a leg curl with an elastic toner necessitates securing the end of the toner to your foot. Once this is achieved,

Leg Curl Machine Start

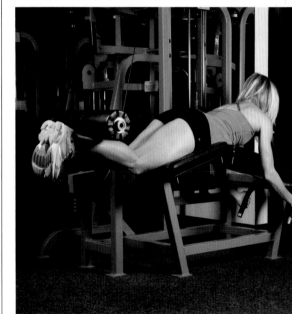

Leg Curl Machine Finish

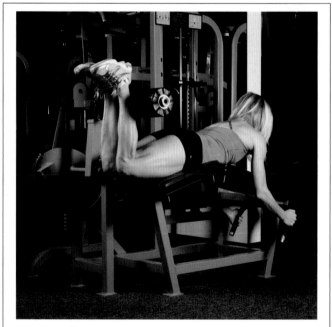

- Lie with your belly on the machine bench, chest flat, and grab the handgrips.

- Place the back of your ankles against the movable pad.

- Adjust pad height as needed.

- Your knees are in line with the rotating cam, which is the pivot point for the mechanical movement.

- Curl legs up, keeping hips down against the bench. Avoid arching your back, as this strains the low back.

- Do not use momentum to swing the weight up; this reduces effectiveness.

- Squeeze at the top before lowering slowly back down. Feet stay flexed.

you can carry on with great progress. If not tethered well, the toner will slip off during the down phase and you may experience frustration.

Female athletes are prone to hamstring tears. They tend to have an imbalance between hamstring and quadriceps strength. A test can be performed to measure this (see Stability Leg Curl section). To self-evaluate your hamstring muscles and determine if there is a discrepancy, watch your form during a curl. Do your toes naturally turn in or out?

If your foot wants to rotate in (toes together), you may have a *stronger medial hamstring* muscle. Correct this by forcing your toes outward during the curl. Weakness in the biceps femoris, coupled with too much strength in the medial hamstring muscle, can cause a "knock-kneed" look.

If your foot rotates out (toes point to the outside) during the curl, you may have *medial hamstring weakness*. Correct this by forcing your toes to point inward during the move. Too much strength in the biceps femoris and weakness in the medial hamstring muscle can cause a "bowlegged" stance.

Elastic Toner Leg Curl Start

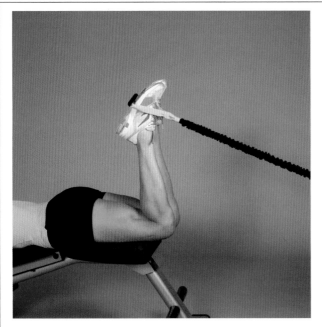

- Anchor the toner low. Place bench so the elastic is taut.

- Lie on your belly with handles placed securely on your feet.

- Position legs in partial curl so toner does not disengage.

Elastic Toner Leg Curl Finish

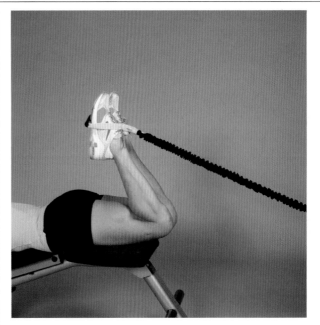

- Curl legs up with fluid movement, keeping hips on the bench. Squeeze at top of the movement before lowering.

- Range of motion may be less than with leg curl

machine due to challenges with keeping toner attached to your foot.

- Point your toes to engage the calf muscles.

STANDING CALF RAISE
Do not misinterpret the following information as a ban against high heels

The calf muscles form the two shapely bulges on the back of the lower leg. High heel shoes, which raise the heel of the foot, tend to give the illusion of longer, slender, and more toned calves. High heels can also cause low backache, shorten the Achilles tendon, and damage the soft tissue that supports the foot (not to mention the blisters, corns, and bun-

ions that can form). If you spend a lot of time in stilettos, use the exercises in this section to offset these risks.

Your Achilles is the tendonous extension of three muscles in your lower leg: the gastrocnemius, soleus, and plantaris. The Achilles begins near the middle of your calf and passes behind your ankle. It is the strongest tendon in the body.

Calf Raise Start

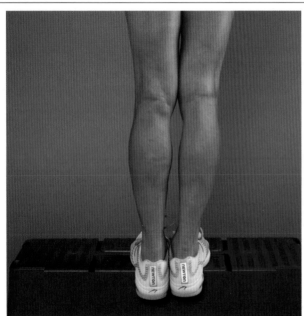

- Stand on a raised step near a wall or handrail. Place the balls of your feet on the edge so heels are free.

- Position legs and feet together; assume neutral body position.

- Drop heels below edge of the step. Do not over-stretch, as this may injure your Achilles.

Calf Raise Finish

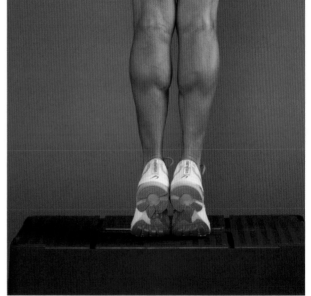

- Lift your heels as high as possible using the calf muscles.

- Pause for a moment at the top. Lower in a controlled motion.

- Modification: Seated calf raises are an easier option.

Nevertheless, jumping around, changing directions, and taking off in a sudden sprint are movements that have been known to pull the Achilles tendon from the calf muscle. You will know if this happens, as it makes a loud pop and causes extreme pain.

Keeping your calf muscles healthy requires TLC of the Achilles tendon. Never force the heel position lower than your normal range of motion. A regular stretching routine, along with strengthening exercises, will prevent you from suffering from a painful Achilles injury. Not to belabor the point, but keeping your Achilles tendon and calf muscles functioning properly is vital.

Achilles tendinitis (which is different from the aforementioned pull) is an inflammation of the tendon, caused from overuse or injury. However, this too is preventable with proper care. If you suffer from this condition, consult your podiatrist about treatment. One treatment surely to be recommended for recovery is eccentric stretching with resistance, more commonly known as calf raises.

Toes Out Calf Raise

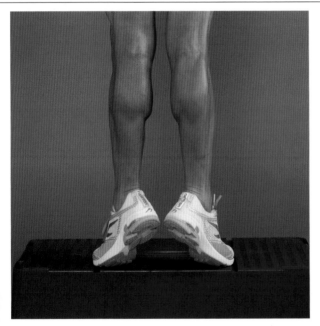

- Use same motion as for calf raise.
- Turn toes out to target the inner, medial head of the gastrocnemius.

Toes In Calf Raise

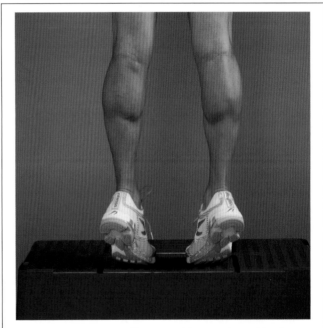

- Use same motion as calf raise.

- Turn toes in to work the lateral and medial heads of the gastrocnemius together.

- The toes-in position has not been proven to isolate the lateral head in the same way the toes-out position isolates the inner medial head.

ONE-LEG, REVERSE CALF RAISE

Flexible muscles and tendons in the lower leg are extremely important for prevention of injury

A group of seven muscles makes up the posterior part of the lower leg. Some muscles are superficial, and some are deeper. The deeper muscles are mostly on the underside of the foot and toe bones and help you point your toes. The superficial muscles are used for movements that involve pushing your heel off the floor, like running, jumping, and dancing.

The upper calf muscle, the gastrocnemius, helps steady your legs when you stand. The lower calf muscle, the soleus, allows you to point your toes and assists the heel lift during mild movements, like walking. Agility sports and functional training require lower leg and ankle strength. A lack of conditioning in the calf muscles, especially the smaller muscles,

One-Leg Calf Raise

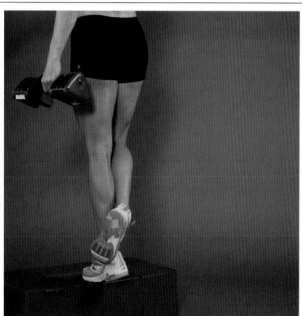

- Stand on a raised step near a wall or handrail (for balance, if needed). Place ball of left foot on the edge so the heel is free.

- Hold a dumbbell with your left hand, palm in. Position right foot behind left heel.

- Raise and lower heel. Do not overstretch in down position.

- Repeat with other leg.

Reverse Calf Raise Start

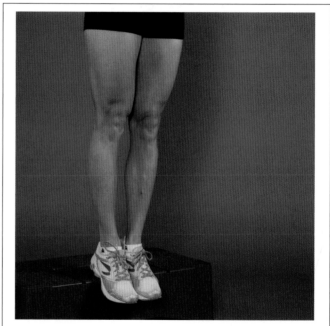

- Shoes with soles that grip are recommended.

- Stand on a raised step. Place your heels on the edge so toes are free.

- Lower forefoot toward the floor.

- This works the muscles in the front of the lower leg.

will reduce your ability to develop optimal physical fitness.

When winter comes around and you venture out for some Nordic or Alpine skiing, you'll be happy you trained the small muscles in your shins, called the tibialis anterior muscles. In the warmer months, inline skating and running are common culprits for fatiguing this muscle. Have you heard of shin splints? This is really an overuse condition believed to be in part a result of muscle weakness. Exercises (such as reverse calf raises) that strengthen the anterior muscles may help alleviate or avoid shin splints.

Reverse Calf Raise Finish

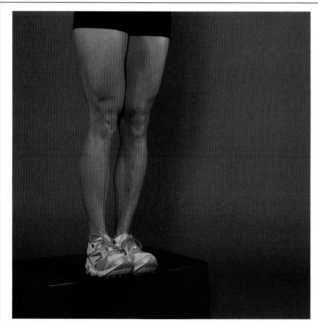

- Pull your forefeet up toward your body as far as possible.
- Flex each foot equally.
- Return by extending your feet until toes point downward.
- Keep knees and hips straight.

GREEN ● LIGHT

If your calf muscles are less than symmetrical, use one-leg dumbbell calf raises to isolate the individual legs. Add a couple of extra reps to the weak or smaller side. If you want to develop more mass overall, standing and seated calf raises are recommended. Seated calf raises are said to give your muscles more cut.

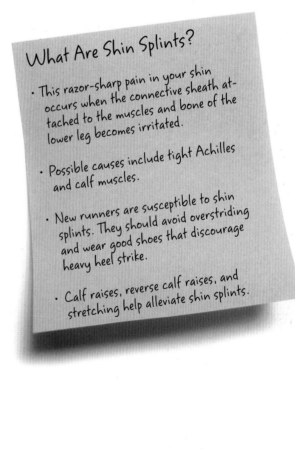

What Are Shin Splints?

- This razor-sharp pain in your shin occurs when the connective sheath attached to the muscles and bone of the lower leg becomes irritated.

- Possible causes include tight Achilles and calf muscles.

- New runners are susceptible to shin splints. They should avoid overstriding and wear good shoes that discourage heavy heel strike.

- Calf raises, reverse calf raises, and stretching help alleviate shin splints.

STANDING FLEX KICK

Dancers have beautiful leg definition, in part from training, but also because they are thin

The time has come to put aside the dumbbells and grab your yoga mat. This chapter is dedicated to moves that sculpt and burn. Ironically, these relatively simple moves tend to burn the most. If it's a dancer's body you're after, time to work the lower muscles from multiple angles.

Standing point exercises are part of the program. Variations

(not shown) include a flat foot stance, a toe stance, turning your toes out, and a straight leg kick out. You can perform a bent knee lift, where you extend the leg out and to the knee repeatedly without touching the floor, or a hopping point move, where one leg stays grounded while you kick the other out in front. When flexing your leg, always point your toe

Forward Kick Start

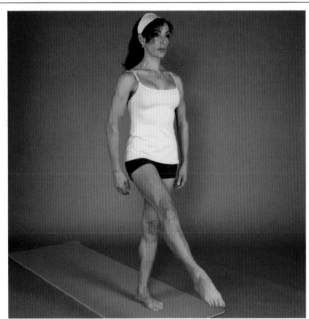

- Stand on the front of a mat in neutral body position, arms at your sides.

- Retract your shoulders and engage your abdominals.

- Extend your right leg forward with toes pointed.

- Keep hips square.

Forward Kick Finish

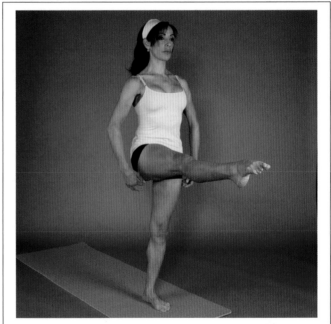

- Keep torso erect, shoulders retracted, and abdominals engaged.

- Lift right leg until it's parallel to the floor or as high as possible without compromising your upper-body position.

- Keep your knee facing up by internally rotating the inner thigh.

- Pulse three times.

to contract the muscles. This alone is a powerful isometric exercise.

Let's clear up a point before continuing. If you're on a weight-loss program, looking to lose body fat, these exercises are not the solution. They will offer many benefits but will not help to increase muscle mass, rev up your metabolism, or create an engine upon which you burn more calories. You should continue compound exercises and strength training, combined with diet and cardio exercise, to achieve your goals.

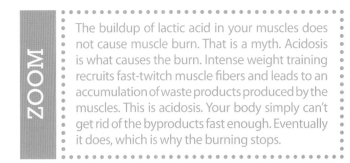
Back Kick Start

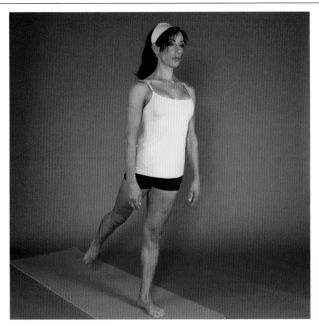

- Lower your right leg and swing it back behind your body in a controlled movement.

- Do not let your hips rotate forward. Keep your pelvis slightly tucked.

- Make sure both legs stay straight and upper body remains erect.

Back Kick Finish

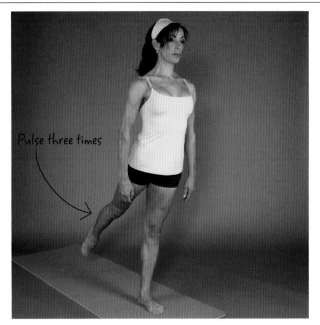

Pulse three times

- Once your right leg is extended behind your body, pause and squeeze the glutes.

- Keep your knee facing down by internally rotating the inner thigh.

- Pulse three times, attempting to lift back leg 1 inch higher with each pulse.

- Repeat with other leg.

DONKEY KICK

Performing this hands-and-knees exercise allows you to target the top of the buttocks

The donkey kick has more than one application. If you are practicing a handstand, the donkey kick is what propels your legs up into the air. Kids love this move. But the donkey kick is not just for kids! What better way to gain fitness and work your glutes than to engage in a playful exercise that makes you feel like a kid again?

When it comes to shaping and lifting your booty, the donkey kick excels. The essence of the exercise is to raise one leg into the air directly behind you, squeezing the buttocks muscles. You can start on your hands and knees or, for a more advanced version, on your hands and feet.

Standing donkey kicks are the more vigorous of the donkey

Donkey Kick: Position 1

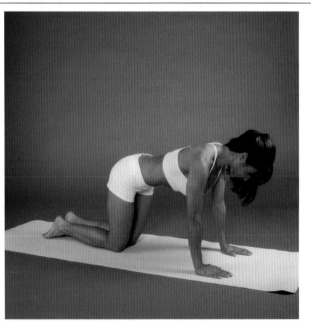

- Start on hands and knees with hips and shoulders square.

- Use neutral spine position, keeping a natural arch to the low back. Retract

shoulders and engage abdominals.

- To avoid placing too much pressure on the kneecaps, press into your shins and feet.

Donkey Kick: Position 2

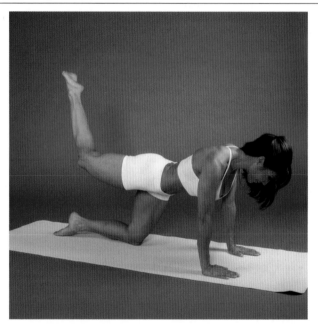

- Continue engaging abdominals. Lift right leg off the mat, keeping your knee bent, and raise foot toward the ceiling in a controlled motion.

- Initiate movement from the

hip, keeping your right leg in a fixed position.

- Don't overarch your back.

- Balance body weight among the three points of contact.

kick exercises and employ a straight leg kick and handstand (not shown). Although you won't formally be in a full, upright handstand, the semi-inverted position requires upper-body strength, balance, and concentration. Inversions are not recommended if you suffer from headaches, heart problems, or high blood pressure.

The more universal donkey kick exercise is the hands-and-knees form described below. However, if you want to kick up your heels and try the straight-leg version, start in a down-dog-ish position. Be sure to employ proper neutral spine posture. Place your palms on the floor about 3 feet in front of your toes. While on your tiptoes, extend one leg into the air behind you. Bend your other knee, push off with that foot, and kick up. Swing legs up and back down to the floor in a straight-leg scissors move. After a few minutes, your heart rate will increase, and your flexibility will improve; providing increased enjoyment and fluidity.

Donkey Kick: Position 3

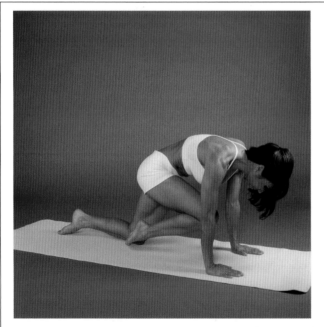

- Tuck your right knee into your chest, keeping shoulders stationary and arms straight.

- Contract your abdominals as knee comes forward. Drop head slightly and round your back to intensify the crunch.

- Do not rotate your hips during the movement.

- Variation: Balance on a BOSU with knees and hands.

Donkey Kick: Position 4

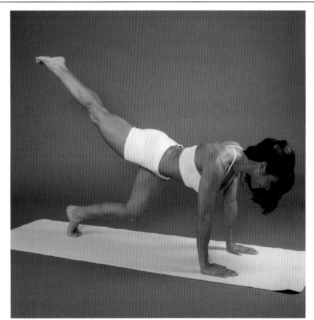

- Release the crunch, retract shoulders, and engage abdominals.

- Extend right leg behind your body while lifting onto your left toes. Lengthen the spine and keep hips square.

- Repeat on other side.

- This final move can be performed as a stand-alone exercise.

KNEELING SIDE KICK

Fire hydrants may be a male dog's latrine, but they're also a toning tool for the tush

The kneeling side kick, also called the fire hydrant, is an exercise popularized in the 1980s. Its purpose was to give you "Buns of Steel." The fire hydrant mimics the movement male dogs use to urinate, thus the name. This movement activates hip, thigh, buttock, and hamstring muscles.

The fire hydrant also helps you maintain functionality to the hip and groin area. Lateral leg lifts open the hips and improve range of motion. It is one of many simple drills that can enrich your muscle patterns, which crosses over to athletics and daily activity.

Perform fire hydrants with steady, controlled movements. If you have tight hips, you may only be able to lift your knee

Kneeling Side Kick: Position 1

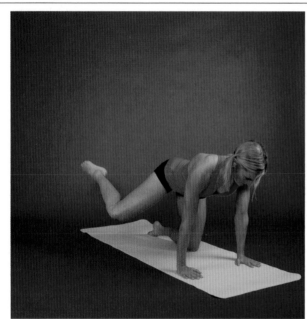

- Start on hands and knees with hips and shoulders square.

- Raise right leg to the side, keeping knee at a 90-degree angle.

- Keep torso parallel to the floor during the movement. If hip rotates with leg, you've got some stretching to do!

Kneeling Side Kick: Position 2

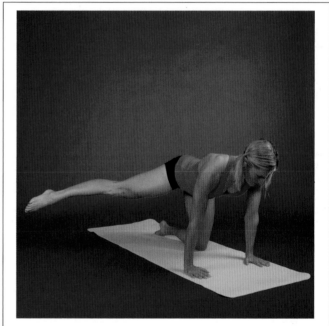

- While maintaining upper body position, straighten right leg to the side of your body.

- Point toes and flex your leg. Keep knee facing forward

- by externally rotating the thigh.

- Hold position for a moment.

15 degrees while keeping the hips parallel to the floor. Raising your leg farther than your hip mobility allows can lead to cramping and is not proper form.

Here are other drills that benefit the hips and groin. Do these at work, in airports, and when you feel the need to loosen up. Find a wall. Do each leg swing ten times on both sides.

Back and forth: Stand with side to wall, place one hand on wall for support. Swing opposite leg forward and backward.

In and out: Stand facing wall farther than arm distance away. Lean forward and place both hands on the wall. Swing one leg out to the side and back across.

In, out, and hold: Same as in and out, just hold leg for a few seconds during highest outer swing and hold it a few seconds during inner swing.

Hip flex and extend: Stand facing wall farther than arm distance away. Lean forward and place both hands on wall. With toes lifted, pull one knee up to chest. Hold. Using your hip, kick leg behind you as far as possible.

Kneeling Side Kick: Position 3

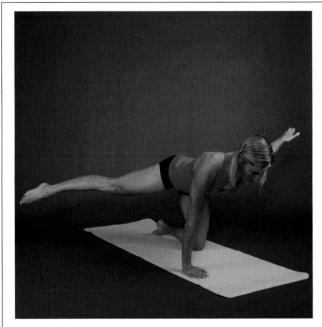

- Neck and spine remain in alignment.

- Activate your core by engaging abdominals and raise left arm to the side of your body.

- Keep torso still while lengthening your right leg and left arm.

- Repeat on other side.

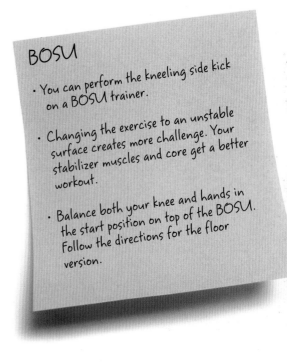

BOSU

• You can perform the kneeling side kick on a BOSU trainer.

• Changing the exercise to an unstable surface creates more challenge. Your stabilizer muscles and core get a better workout.

• Balance both your knee and hands in the start position on top of the BOSU. Follow the directions for the floor version.

INNER, OUTER THIGH

Workouts are more effective if you focus on and visualize the muscles you are targeting

Always know what muscles you are training. Throughout you have been given information on where muscles are in your body and how they perform. This was done for a reason. Visualization is a powerful transformational tool. Can you picture what muscle you are working? How do you want that muscle to perform? What are you doing mentally to make it happen?

"If the *why* is big enough, the *how to* will come." That is a quote from a motivational speaker named Randy Gage. It is simple, yet profound. When performing an exercise, you might let your mind wander and hope the set ends quickly. Or, you can spend the moment focusing on proper form, concentrating on your body's alignment, and visualizing the

Inner Thigh Toning Start

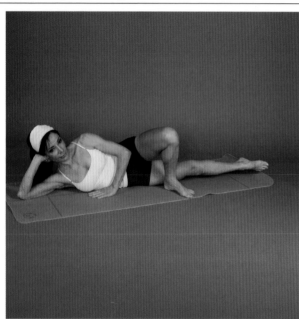

- Lie on your right side with head resting in right palm.

- Cross your left foot in front of your right leg, kneecap facing the ceiling.

- Place your left palm on the mat in front of your chest.

- Extend your right leg long, lengthening your body.

Inner Thigh Toning Finish

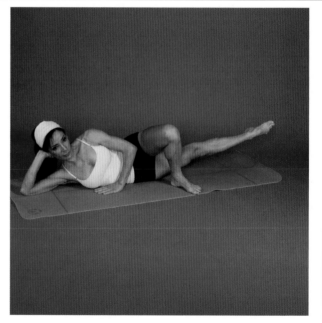

- Raise your right leg, using the inner thigh muscles.

- Turn the right heel slightly toward the ceiling.

- Place emphasis on the lifting movement, using small pulses.

- Repeat on other side.

overall contribution each perfect repetition makes to your health and well-being.

The adductor, or inner thigh muscle, has fibers that are short and horizontal. It also has fibers that are directed laterally and downward. When performing inner-thigh work, focus on stretching and elongating the muscle. This visualization is not about the fat that may be resting on top of the muscle; it needs to be about the muscle itself. You will surely feel the precise spot once you start moving!

Inner-Outer Thigh Toning Start

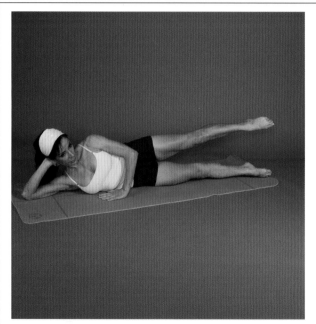

- Lie on your right side with head resting in right palm and both legs extended.

- Place left palm on the mat in front of your chest.

- Stabilize your torso and press hip into the mat.

- Raise your left leg by contracting the outer thigh. Do not rotate the knee.

Inner-Outer Thigh Toning Finish

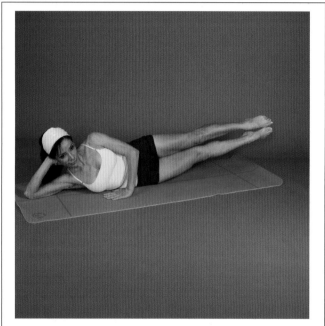

- Hold upper body still by engaging your abdominals. Do not sink into the shoulders.

- Raise your right leg to meet the left leg by contracting the inner thigh muscles.

- If your hip pops, readjust leg position and squeeze buttocks.

- Repeat on other side.

MOVES THAT SCULPT

165

SIDE-LYING KICK

Rond de jambe is a ballet term that literally means "circle of the leg"

Having something to hold on to equates with assistance. There's a reason handrails are required code on stairways. They help with balance and provide stability.

The young rarely use handrails. Actually, the very young do, but only because Mom tells them to. A child's instinct is to barrel down the steps. Healthy, strong adolescents have an enormous amount of confidence and ability. They skip steps. On the other hand, out-of-shape and overweight adults move deliberately and hold tightly to any object that will help them along. Which state of being is preferable?

Keeping your body agile requires pushing it through a complete repertoire of positions and actions. You can accomplish this by letting go of the banister and asking more from your muscles. Instead of pushing off the sides of your chair when getting up, for example, why not use your core and leg strength to rise free of assistance.

Grand Rond de Jambe: Position 1

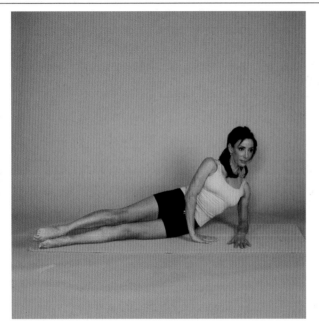

- Lie on your left side with elbow at 90 degrees. Lengthen the back of the neck by pressing the crown of your head away from shoulders.

- Don't let ribs sink into the mat.

- Position legs at a 45-degree angle in front of your body.

- Extend legs equally long.

Grand Rond de Jambe: Position 2

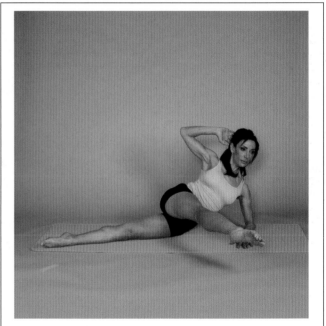

- Maintain upper-body position and place right hand behind ear, elbow to side.

- Swing your right leg in front of your body, initiating movement from the hip.

- Focus on your right leg, keeping left hip pressed into the mat.

- Continue lengthening the spine.

When performing floor exercises, such as *Rond de jambe*, practice the same theory. Instead of leaning excessively on your arm for balance, use more core strength and total body muscle activation to hold your position. Unassisted movement may be the solution to incorporating more balance into your life.

Grand Rond de Jambe: Position 3

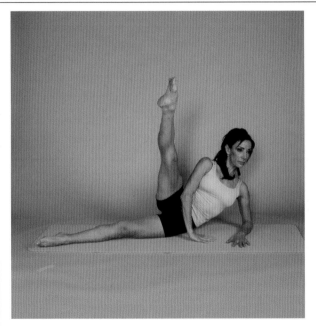

- Bring right palm back to mat in front of your body.

- Swing right foot up toward the ceiling by rotating leg in hip socket.

- Don't let ribs sink into the mat.

- Keep pressing shoulders down away from ears.

Grand Rond de Jambe: Position 4

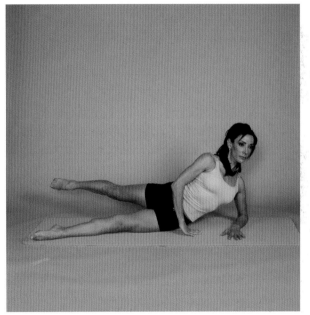

- Lower your right leg and extend it behind your body.

- Press right hip forward. Stretch upper back to counterbalance against the weight of your right leg as it extends back.

- Repeat with other side.

- Variation: Reverse the sequence.

MOVES THAT SCULPT

LUNGE AND SIDE KICK

The resistance becomes more difficult as you go further into the lunge with elastic toners

Elastic toners are a practical method of training. The portability alone makes them a perfect accessory on an overnight trip. Functional fitness has made toners more popular than ever.

It used to be that the only time you were handed a piece of rubber exercise tubing was when a physical therapist incorporated it into rehabilitation exercises. Today they are well-

designed pieces of equipment. The tubing is an extremely adaptable form of exercise.

Virtually every muscle in the body can be targeted with elastic toners. Doing lunges with them improves strength by increasing the level of difficulty throughout the motion. Preloading the toner increases the resistance for a harder

Elastic Toner Lunge Start

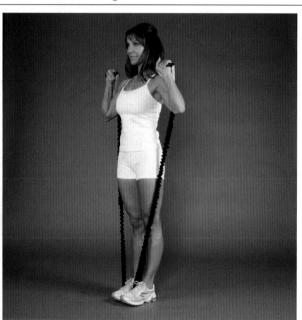

- Place toner under your right foot and stand in neutral body position.

- Hold handles over your shoulders to create tension in the elastic.

- Retract shoulders and engage abdominals.

Elastic Toner Lunge Finish

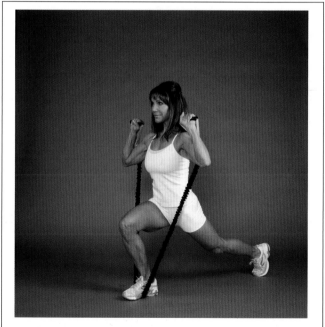

- Perform a reverse lunge with your left leg. Do not let your knee touch the floor.

- Keep upper body erect and elastic taut.

- From this position, perform static lunges up and down.

- Repeat on other side.

workout. Watch how you can reeducate and strengthen your muscles and increase endurance.

A fairly new concept with manufacturers like Oxygenfit is to color code the handles. This is meant to be appealing to women. And, frankly, it is. If yours are not color coded, fear not.

When purchasing new elastic toners, look for a comfortable handle and a safety sleeve over the elastic. This helps eliminate overstretching and wear and tear. It's been mentioned before, but a door anchor attachment is the only way you can easily accommodate a maximum number of exercises.

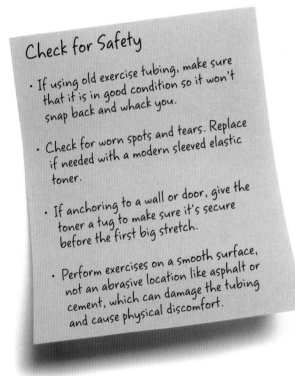
ZOOM

Sleeved elastic toners are available in a range of colors that relate to their resistance. The pastel version uses *Pearl* (very light), *Blush* (light), *Sky* (medium), *Silver* (heavy), and *Black* (very heavy). If you train in a gym, resistance bands typically are *Yellow* (thin), *Red* (medium), *Green* (heavy), *Blue* (extra heavy), *Black* (special heavy), and *Silver* (super heavy).

Elastic Toner Side Kick

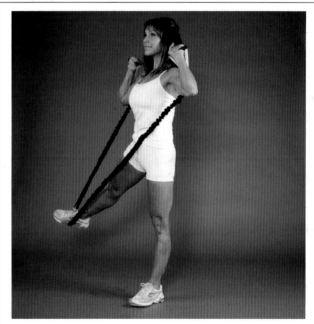

- This is a hip-opening exercise.

- Place band under your right foot and stand in neutral body position.

- Raise leg to the side, allowing elastic toner to assist with lift. Keep hips square.

- Toners with greater resistance offer more assistance.

MOVES THAT SCULPT

169

INVIGORATING STRETCHES

Invigorate means to impart strength and vitality; to be invigorated is to be alive and animated

A few invigorating stretches can help open up your body, channel your energy, and make you feel alive. The prayer twist and seated spine stretch are postures that increase flexibility in the lower back and hips. They also improve tone in the abdominals, hips, and buttocks. A spinal twist even soothes away tension in your upper back and shoulders.

Another benefit of twisting happens deep on the inside of your body. Twisting simultaneously stretches and contracts the muscles in the back and abdomen. This causes a compression of the spine, improving blood flow and circulation. The internal organs end up getting a massage of their own, which improves digestion.

Side Prayer Twist

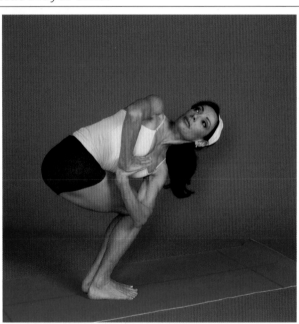

- Stand with feet and legs together. Bend forward and come to a 45-degree squat.

- With hands at heart, rotate upper body, bringing left elbow outside of right thigh.

- Lengthen your spine and neck. Keep knees and hips square.

- Turn head toward ceiling.

- Repeat on other side.

Seated Spine Stretch

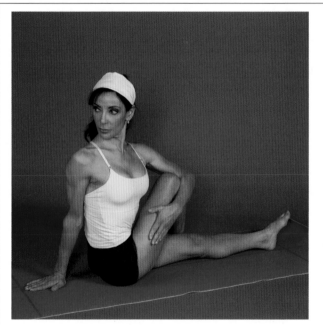

- Sit with tall spine and legs extended.

- Cross right foot over left leg.

- Plant right hand behind your body. Lift your chest and rotate your torso,

- bringing your left arm over right knee.

- Keep hips on the mat and look over your right shoulder.

- Repeat on other side.

Cobra pose is named after the serpent of the same name. It is also a means of strengthening the back and abdominals. Like twisting-spine poses, the cobra pose provides stimulation to the internal organs, aiding in digestion. As you expand your chest with breath, your body becomes alive with energy.

The plough exercise is a wonderful pose for stretching the back, neck, hamstrings, and shoulders. This pose can place undue weight on the upper neck, specifically the cervical and thoracic areas. It may therefore be inappropriate if you have arthritis or osteoporosis of the spine.

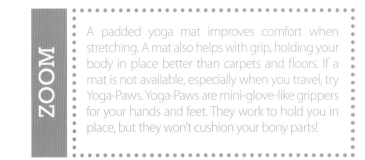
Gentle Cobra

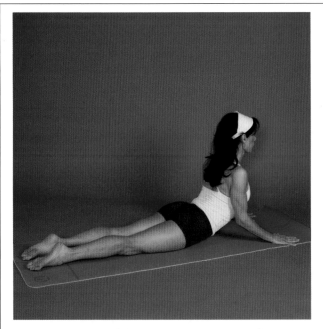

- Lie on your belly with legs extended. Place palms at sides at chest level.

- Press hips and thighs into the mat and lift your chest off the mat, keeping elbows close to your body.

- Maintain space between your shoulders and ears by sliding shoulder blades down your back.

Plough

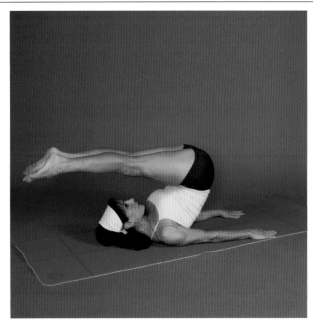

- Lie on your back with legs together and palms facing down.

- Engage abdominals and lift legs toward the ceiling. Continue by lifting hips off the floor one vertebra at a time.

- Send your legs over top of your head. Do not fold chin into chest.

TEN-MINUTE TUNE-UP

COMPOUND ABS

When's the last time you heard someone say, "I just wasted ten minutes getting fit?"

If you have only ten precious minutes of time to squeeze in a workout, do it. It won't be for naught. It is true that you should aim for longer sessions, but please do yourself a favor and keep consistent. Stopping and starting an exercise program will stifle momentum. You are on a lifelong training program that is meant to add value to your years, not over-whelm you with more responsibility. It is a matter of perspective and priorities.

The paradox is this: If you are truly injured or sick with the most unfortunate of situations, be it cancer, paralysis, or other life-changing circumstances, the very thing you want to do is exercise. You will begin to crave moving. You will yearn

Drop Arm Start

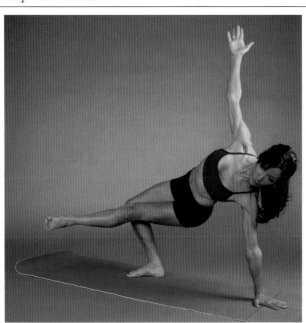

- This is an advanced move.

- Start in a left-side plank position.

- Place right foot on the mat, behind the left knee.

- Extend right arm to the ceiling and lift your left leg off mat.

- Retract shoulders and engage abdominals.

Drop Arm Finish

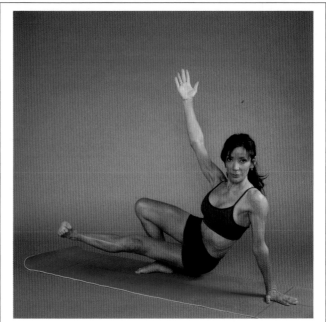

- Maintain overall strength.

- Keep right arm and left leg lifted, drop hips straight toward the mat, contracting your obliques.

- Lift hips back to start

position. Keep right and left arms in alignment.

- To relieve pressure on the wrists, press through the ball of your hand.

- Repeat on other side.

for life. Even with a broken bone, people can't sit still long enough for it to heal. Whatever your ailment, make use of your body as it allows and celebrate what it offers you.

From the words of Tara Llanes, world champion mountain bike racer who suffered a spinal cord injury and is unable to move her legs, "*Never give up*." Every day she strives to do a little bit more than the day before with the goal of walking again.

Inspiration aside, it's time to prepare yourself for a set of heart-pumping abdominal exercises. These are much bet-ter than ten minutes of crunches, because they work your entire body. The obliques, lower back, glutes, and thighs get pumped along with the arms, legs, neck, hands, and feet. The compound drop arm exercise and the straight leg side crunch engage ten times more muscle mass than just your rectus abdominis alone. In ten minutes you're doing the equivalent of over an hour of straight crunches.

Straight Leg Side Crunch Start

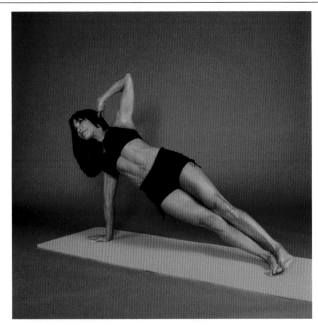

- Start in right-side plank position and place left hand behind left ear, elbow to the side.

- Maintain neutral body position. Retract shoulders and engage abdominals.

- Don't let hips sink into mat.

Straight Leg Side Crunch Finish

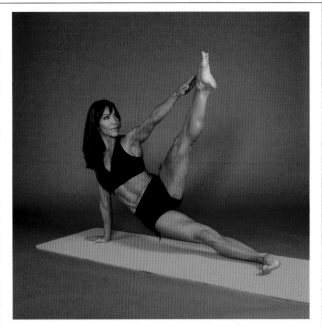

- Press your right foot into the mat while extending your left leg toward the ceiling.

- Reach left arm up and to-ward the toes, maintaining lengthened spine.

- Turn head to face your left hand. Activate your core to avoid toppling sideways.

PUSH-UPS, SHOULDER BRIDGE

Leave prodigious feats of strength to Olympians and focus on your own pound-for-pound strength

Knowing your relative strength capabilities can help you decide which exercises to do. A wall push-up (not shown) is much easier than a decline push-up. If you are fit and have a very high strength-to-weight ratio, go for the challenge. If you are overweight or deconditioned, start with the basics.

Strength-to-weight ratio, also called specific strength, is a measure of a material's strength divided by its weight. This is best illustrated by the materials used on airplanes, which need to be very strong yet very light. In human terms, strength-to-weight ratio has to do with strength relative to body weight. Some people still cling to the myth that bigger means stronger, but this is often not true. When an exercise

One-Leg Decline Push-up

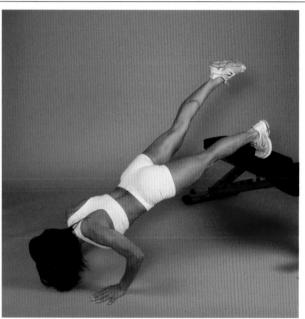

- Place your toes on a bench and hands shoulder-width apart on the floor.

- Retract shoulders and, with hips and waist straight, engage abdominals.

- Lift your right leg off the bench. Keep hips straight. Perform push-ups.

- Repeat on other leg.

High-Low Push-up

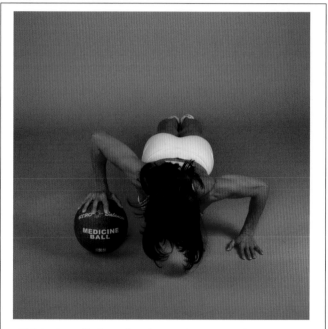

- This is also called simulated one-arm push-up.

- Assume push-up position on the floor and place your right hand on top of a medicine ball. Perform push-ups.

- Repeat on other arm.

- Modifications: For easier options, place knees on floor; use push-up handle instead of ball.

involves gravity, being small, light, and strong is advantageous over the brute force of volume.

This is important when doing body-weight exercises. Changing the angle of an exercise affects how much gravity comes into play, thus altering the amount of body weight being lifted at any given time. For example, a decline push-up is more challenging than a regular push-up. Because the body is tipped downward, the arms and chest support more of the weight. Conversely, an incline push-up is easier, because the legs support more of the weight.

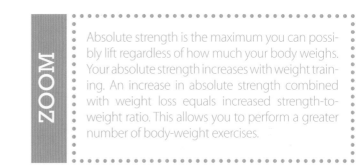

ZOOM

Absolute strength is the maximum you can possibly lift regardless of how much your body weighs. Your absolute strength increases with weight training. An increase in absolute strength combined with weight loss equals increased strength-to-weight ratio. This allows you to perform a greater number of body-weight exercises.

Bridge Start

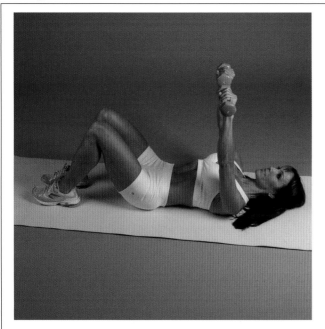

- Lie on your back with knees bent and legs together.

- Use neutral body position. Retract shoulders and engage abdominals.

- Lift dumbbells over your chest with straight arms and overhand grip.

- Do not lock your elbows.

Bridge Finish

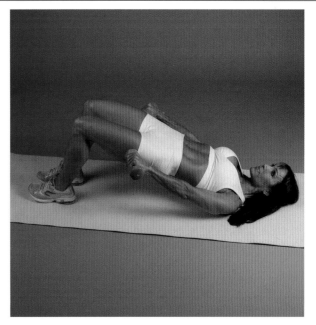

- Lift hips and come into a bridge position. Simultaneously lower your arms to the sides.

- Keep pelvis slightly tucked and use inner thigh muscles

- to prevent knees from bowing out.

- Maintain knee, hip, and shoulder alignment.

- Return to start position.

ARC-SQUAT KICK

Allow your leg to travel in a smooth, continuous shape like a curve or an arch

If you have ever taken a cardio kickboxing class, you'll understand the power of a kick. These classes are rigorous. A long warm-up is required to get the legs ready for a strike. Kicking builds stamina and burns calories, especially when combined with other compound movements.

Take it from those who have adopted kick training into their fitness program: A little goes a long way. Ten minutes will give you just the tune-up you're looking for to break a sweat. The key to making this an effective move is to control your pace.

Overextending yourself by squatting too deep or kicking too high on the first round will detour your objective. Always

Arc-Squat Kick: Position 1

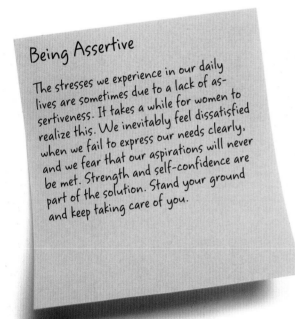

- Stand in neutral body position and come into a sumo squat (plié squat).

- Perform a roundhouse kick with your right leg by swinging the leg across your body and around to the right side.

- Engage abdominals to stabilize the upper body.

watch that you don't lock a joint when kicking. The last thing you want to do is pull a muscle or tendon.

It is probably best to avoid any kicking if you're just off a long airplane flight and your legs have been cramped for an extended period of time. However, if you're sufficiently limber and warm, try the arc-squat kick. Repetition of this move for ten minutes helps with focus, sharpens reflexes, and improves technique.

Arc-Squat Kick: Position 2

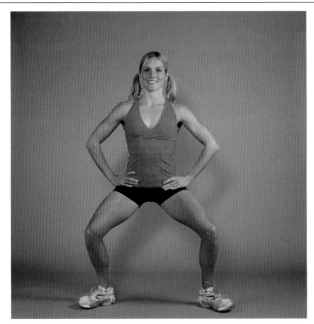

- Finish the roundhouse kick by returning to sumo squat position.
- Keep hands on hips and head up throughout the movement.
- Torso remains in frontal plane.

Arc-Squat Kick: Position 3

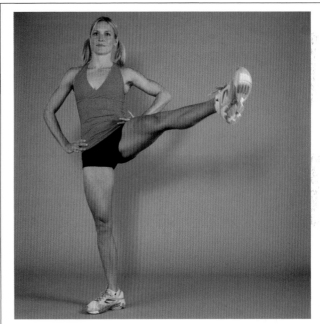

- Perform roundhouse kick with your left leg by swinging the leg across your body and around to the left side.
- Turn toes slightly out to focus on the inner thighs and decrease tension on the quads.
- Focus on kicking at the same height with each leg.

177

REVERSE PLANK
No matter what your age, you need to take care of your knees

Knee pain is common for women. If you suffer when you walk up and down stairs or stand up from a chair, or if it hurts to squat or kneel, you may be suffering from chondromalacia patellae, also known as patellofemoral pain syndrome. *Runner's knee* is another term to describe the snapping, popping, or grinding in the patellar region.

The causes of the condition are varied. Chondromalacia is often associated with overuse or misalignment in the knee.

Misalignment can be the result of tight muscles or tendons, which pull the patella off-track, or the result of genetics in the way your hips, legs, knees, and feet align. Other orthopedic doctors believe patellofemoral syndrome may be caused by a type of softening within the tissues under the kneecap.

Professional athletes and dancers are not immune to knee pain. Many suffer through the pain and continue to train. This is not a good idea. The longer symptoms persist, the more

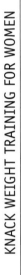

Reverse Plank: Position 1

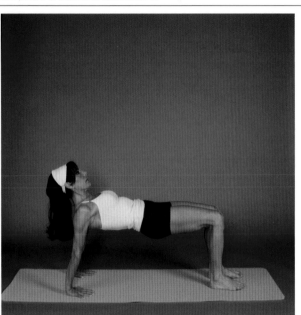

- Sit on a mat with knees bent, feet flat. Place hands behind hips, fingers and toes pointing in the same direction.

- Lift hips into modified reverse plank until torso

- is parallel to the floor and knees are at 90 degrees.

- Arms are perpendicular to the floor and chest is lifted.

Reverse Plank: Position 2

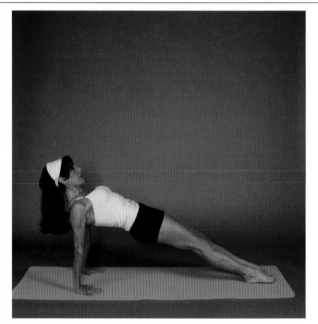

- Maintain arm position and keep chest lifted.

- Extend legs straight, keeping inner thighs together.

- Body is aligned from shoulders to ankles.

- Keep head slightly forward to decrease tension on neck.

inflamed the joint becomes, and then a longer recovery period is needed.

Recommended exercises to help prevent knee pain include the reverse plank, which strengthens the muscles in the legs. Remember to keep your muscles and tendons pliable and flexible as part of your pain-free program. Master the ability to hold a straight leg reverse plank for one minute before progressing to the one-leg version.

Reverse Plank: Position 3

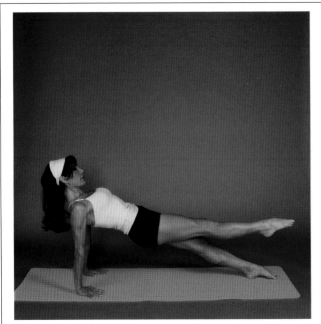

- While maintaining reverse-plank position, engage abdominals and lift your right leg off the mat with toes pointed.

- Do not let hips drop during the movement. Take pressure off your wrists by pressing actively into your left foot.

- Keep hips square.

Reverse Plank: Position 4

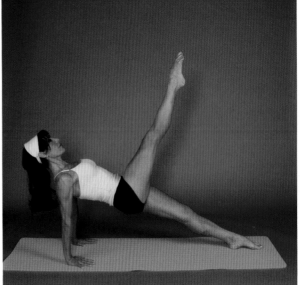

- Kick your right leg straight up as high as possible.

- Keep hips elevated and square. Do not sink into your shoulders.

- Flex your foot to return to start position.

- Repeat on other leg.

YOGA POSTURES 1

In Vinyasa-style yoga, poses should flow from one to another in conjunction with the breath

Vinyasa (pronounced *vin-yaah-sa*) is a Sanskrit term used in relation to certain styles of yoga. It is a flowing, dynamic form of yoga in which attention is placed on the journey between multiple postures, not just the individual postures themselves. A standard *vinyasa* consists of the flow from commonly practiced postures like plank, to low plank, to upward-facing dog,

to downward-facing dog. The purpose of *vinyasa* is to create heat in the body, which leads to purification through increased circulation and sweating. It also improves flexibility, as well as tendon strength.

Asana is the Sanskrit term for a particular body position primarily intended to restore and maintain well-being, improve

Downward-Facing Dog

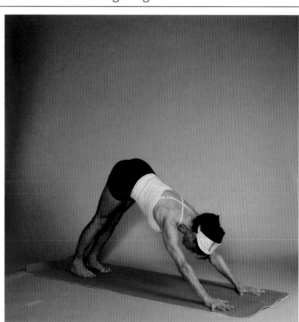

- Start on hands and knees.

- Spread your fingers, fold toes under, and lift hips toward the ceiling, extending the arms and legs.

- Press back into your heels.

Slide shoulder blades down and back. Press index finger joints into the mat and lengthen your inner arms.

Downward-Facing Dog Split Pose

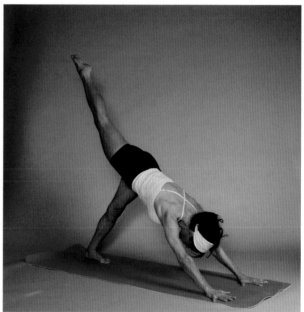

- Keep your belly lifted away from your arms to relieve pressure on the wrists.

- Lengthen your neck and continue retracting shoulders.

- Lift your right leg until it is aligned with your body. Keep hips square.

- Rotate your inner thigh so knee faces the floor.

the body's flexibility, and promote vitality. Asanas today encompass a variety of lying and standing positions, which differs from the original practice of prolonged meditative sitting postures. *Ashtanga vinyasa* yoga is a distinct practice that incorporates the physical movement with Buddhist philosophy. The practice is based on eight (*ashta*) limbs (*anga*) of classical yoga. The limbs, or yoga sutras, are based on the influence of Buddha's Noble Eightfold paths. The path is an instrument of discovery to gradually generate insights unveiling the ultimate truth of things. Being on the right path

denotes completion, togetherness, and coherence. Asanas, therefore, should be steady and comfortable, firm yet relaxed.

The poses shown here provide a basis upon which to start developing your personal practice. Further your study and establish your own spiritual journey with an *ashtanga vinyasa* yoga sequence. You might begin with ten Sun Salutations and the standing poses. Next, move to a back-bending sequence. Finally, finish with a set of inverted postures. Seek out a yoga class in your area for more information.

Forward Lunge

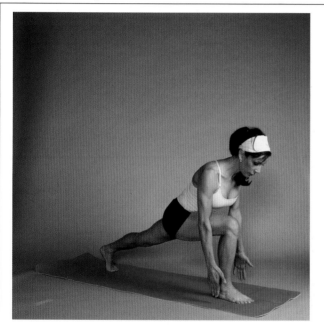

- Bring right leg forward and come into a forward lunge, toes of both feet facing forward. With neutral spine, lengthen from crown of the head.

- Avoid sinking into your hips by engaging your core. Keep knee aligned with ankle, behind the toes.

- Extend through the back of your left foot.

Crescent Lunge

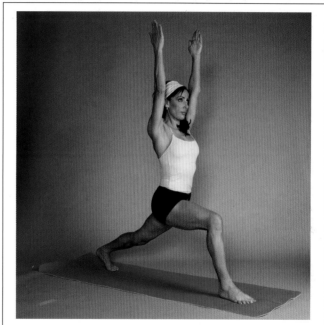

- Without moving your feet or breaking alignment of the knees and ankles, engage abdominals and lift torso.

- Bring arms above your head, palms facing each other. Retract your shoulders and tuck tailbone slightly.

- Sink deeper into the lunge and lengthen the spine.

- Repeat sequence on other side.

YOGA POSTURES 2

Yoga has evolved (or devolved) into a form of exercise in the United States

Yoga dates back over five thousand years. While it is a spiritual practice in India, it has evolved into a lucrative business in the United States. *Yoga Journal* magazine reports that about 16.5 million Americans spend nearly $3 billion annually on classes and products. Many purists would classify this as devolution, not progress.

Today you can find a variety of off-beat yoga practices. These classes may appeal to the practitioner who is unwilling, uninterested, or unable to reach a level of advanced self-enlightenment. Many of the intangible benefits do carry over, however.

Yoga calms the nervous system and balances the mind,

Warrior II

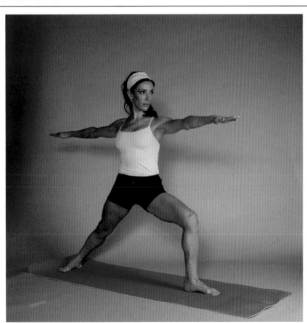

- Come into a forward lunge with left toes forward and right foot turned out.

- Extend left arm forward and right arm back, parallel to the floor, palms down.

- Open your hip and extend your right leg. Keep reaching through the fingertips.

- Retract shoulders, lengthen spine, and gaze over your left arm.

Triangle

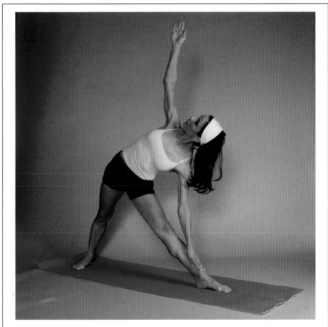

- From Warrior II, straighten left leg.

- Shift hips toward right leg and bend sideways over left leg. All movement is in frontal plane.

- Rest your left hand on your shin, stretch right arm up, and look to the ceiling, twisting at the torso.

body, and spirit. It is believed that those who practice yoga can prevent specific diseases and maladies by keeping the energy meridians open and filled with life energy. Yoga can lower blood pressure and reduce stress.

Yoga's ability to improve concentration, coordination, and flexibility is clear. Just try standing on one leg, extending the other to the side, and grabbing your big toe. There is nothing else in the world you are capable of thinking of in that moment but staying balanced and managing the task at hand.

If you are curious, seek out restorative yoga practices, which encourage a very relaxed state and use props instead of muscular tension to maintain pose alignments. The props help you to move your body in many directions. This is helpful if you have chronic stress or physical limitations.

Inverted poses are beneficial for reversing gravity. Because we sit so much, blood and lymph fluid accumulate in the lower extremities. Being upside down allows fluids to flow in the other direction. This enhances heart function and allows the exchange of oxygen and waste products across the cell membranes.

Half Moon

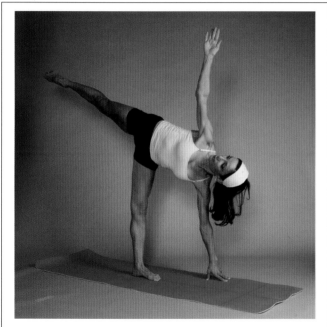

- From Triangle pose, shift weight onto your left leg and left hand.

- Raise right leg in frontal plane until aligned with body. Open the hips.

- Keep ribs facing forward and lift from the sternum, or breastbone.

- Lengthen arms and turn head toward ceiling.

Standing Forward Bend

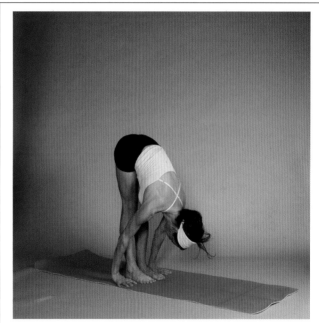

- From Half Moon pose, bring right leg and right hand back to the floor in a controlled movement.

- Bend forward from the hips. Focus on lengthening your torso, pressing heels into the floor and lifting the sit bones. Let your head hang.

- Roll up one vertebra at a time.

- Repeat sequence on other side.

PUSH-UP TO PIKE

It's time to enhance your ability in all tasks that involve physical competency

Functional fitness exercises provide the extra edge of efficiency that can mean the difference between slipping and falling. Developing unconscious competence is the ultimate endpoint of motor recruitment patterns. This is the ability to perform tasks without having to think about them.

Putting one foot in front of the other when you walk is an

automatic pattern. Eventually sitting on a stability ball will be one, too. Remember perfect practice makes perfect. You can train the motor paths to perform at a higher level and become part of your unconscious competence, but it takes time, effort, and consistency.

The combination of physical strength, greater balance, core

Push-up to Pike: Position 1

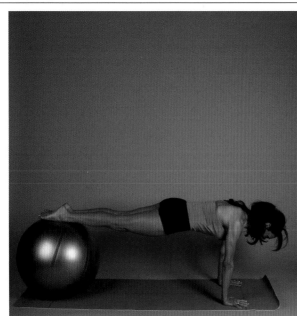

- Position belly or shins on a ball and hands on the floor.

- Walk hands forward until your ankles are on top of the ball.

- Maintain straight body alignment from head to feet.

- Support your upper body with extended arms, shoulder-width apart.

Push-up to Pike: Position 2

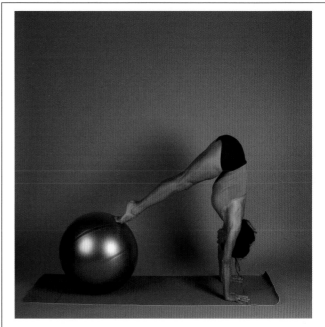

- Retract shoulders and engage abdominals.

- Come into a handstand pike position by pressing your back up and lifting hips toward the ceiling. Roll the ball with your legs until

- your toes are barely touching the ball.

- Keep pressing hands into the mat and maintain vertical upper-body alignment.

stability, and cat-like reflexes translates into the ability to dodge that fast-moving object and walk over an icy sidewalk with confidence. Always use good judgment and do what you can to avoid a potential hazard. But be prepared for the unexpected.

Strive to keep your muscles supple. Supple muscles are capable of bending and twisting with ease. Movement is fluid and without stiffness. Healthy muscle tissue is compliant and readily adaptable or responsive to new situations. The push-up to pike exercise is synonymous with functional competence and a means for keeping your muscles supple

Push-up to Pike: Position 3

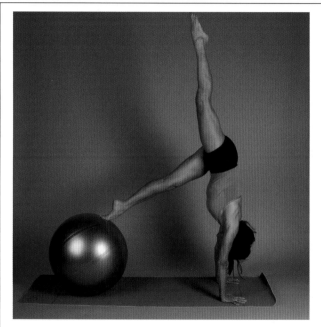

- Keep your upper body still and toes positioned on the edge of the ball.

- Extend your right leg toward the ceiling. Attempt to create one vertical line from the tip of toe, through the body, to the hands.

- Keep hips square, shoulders retracted, and abdominals engaged.

Push-up to Pike: Position 4

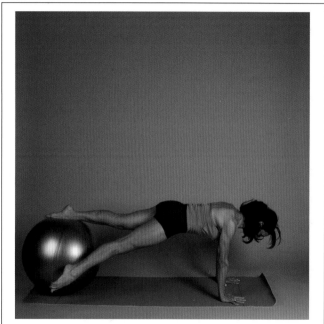

- Slowly lower your right leg to the ball, engage abdominals, straighten legs, and roll back down into a bridge position.

- Without rocking hips, slide right leg off the ball and outline the curve of the ball. Avoid touching the ball.

- Repeat sequence on other side.

185

EXTENSION SEQUENCE

Lordosis behavior refers to the body position some females display when ready to mate

The muscles of the spinal column, along with the core, provide a foundation for bending, squatting, lunging, pushing, pulling, and locomotion. When still, it is these muscles that are responsible for good (or bad) posture.

The spinal column is divided into several geographical regions. Each region includes specific vertebrae referred to by letters and numbers. Starting from the neck, there are the cervical (C1–C7), thoracic (T1–T12), lumbar (L1–L5), and pelvic or sacral (S1–S5) vertebrae and the coccyx, or tailbone.

Lordosis refers to an exaggerated curvature in the lumbar region, or the low back. Lordosis is also an innate mammalian response. Mice, cats, and humans display this behavior when

Advanced Hyperextension

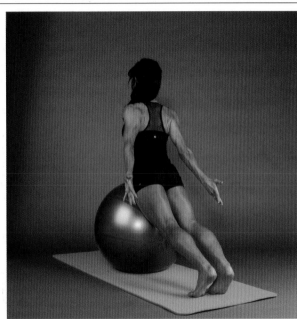

- Lie belly over ball. Straighten legs, placing majority of weight on the pelvis. Plant feet on the mat.

- Squeeze buttocks and raise upper body as high as possible, without overarching.

- Extend arms to sides, palms out. Actively squeeze arms together and lift the chest.

- Slowly lower back so parallel to the floor.

Advanced Reverse Hyperextension

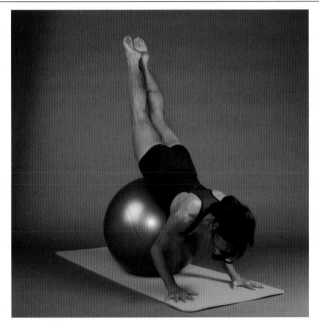

- Lie belly over ball with palms flat on mat. Retract shoulders, engage core, and maintain neutral spine.

- Keeping legs together and straight, lift legs up toward ceiling. Lengthen torso and allow back to arch slightly. Do not fold lower back.

- Keep feet together and squeeze buttocks.

- Slowly lower legs so parallel to floor.

they are ready to mate. They curve their spine so that the apex points in the ventral direction and the hips are elevated, aiding in copulation. Nature never intended this posture to be permanent, so ladies, please tuck your pelvis in during the day.

Sex aside, pregnant women and people with excessive visceral fat may also suffer from lordosis due to the excess weight pulling forward. Tight low-back muscles, weak abdominals, tight quads and hip flexors, and weak hamstrings can also cause lordosis. Lordosis leads to painful spinal injuries and can cause moderate to severe lower back pain.

Oblique Pull-ins

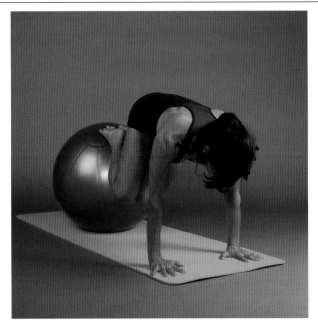

- This exercise is also called jackknife.

- Start in push-up plank position. Roll ball forward by bringing your knees under your hips and toward the right elbow.

- Rotate torso and flatten back slightly to accommodate oblique contraction.

- Repeat on other side.

Lateral Side Flexion

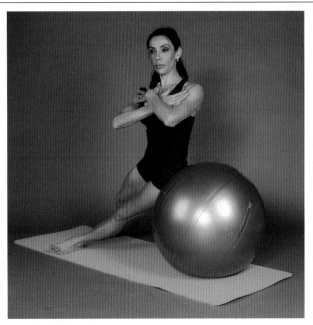

- Place feet at junction of the wall or plant on the mat. Lean your left hip on the ball. Start with torso upright, hands over chest.

- Curl upper body over the ball and continue flexing laterally.

- Repeat on other side.

- Variations: Hold weight. Stretch hands overhead.

BALL BALANCE

Kneeling on a stability ball engages the abdominals and tones the inner thighs

In biomechanics, balance is the ability to maintain your center of gravity with minimal postural sway. Equilibrioception is your sense of balance. Standing on one foot is harder with your eyes closed. Having an inner-ear infection can cause dizziness and disorientation. The common cold can give you vertigo.

You need all your senses working to their maximum capacity in order to score a perfect ten on the balance beam. It is imperative you have your senses (including common sense) when you attempt to kneel and stand on a stability ball. If you have feeble bones and little muscular integrity, you're at risk of falling and breaking something. Falling off a stabil-

Ball Balance: Position 1

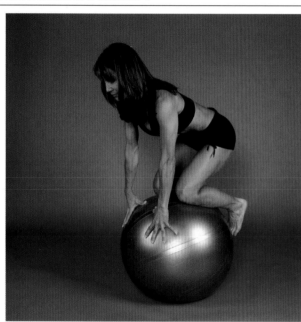

- Place knees and hands on top of the stability ball. Lean forward slightly until your feet come off the floor.

- Engage abdominals and focus eyes forward. Do not look down at the ball.

- Use inner thighs and hands to counterbalance and stabilize.

Ball Balance: Position 2

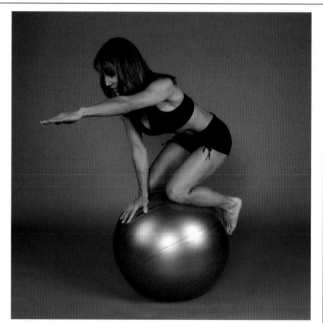

- Slowly and with confidence, raise your upper body slightly and adjust right hand to the center front of the ball.

- Greater core activation means greater stability.

- Lift left arm in front of your body, keeping shoulders retracted.

- Reaching your shoulder out will throw you off balance.

ity ball will slap you to the floor faster than a wipeout on a snowboard.

If you feel your strength and durability are adequate to try these balancing moves, practice a few introductory exercises first. Start with some pelvic tilts, which involve rocking your pelvis forward, backward, and around on the ball. This hip-circling movement gives you a sense of how the ball moves and feels under you.

Next try bouncing. Sit comfortably on the ball and slowly bounce up and down.

Next, grab the ball with your thighs and squeeze while lifting your feet off the floor as you balance. This isometric exercise is a great thigh toner.

Become skilled at complete relaxation on the ball and breathe deeply. Focusing on a point ahead of you helps calm the nerves and maintain balance. Mainly, develop the courage to just climb up and try it.

Ball Balance: Position 3

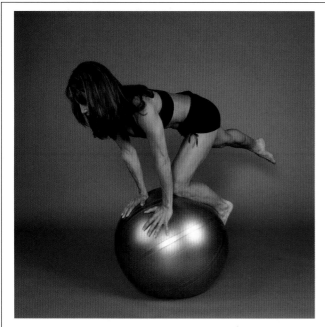

- Reposition your hands back to the top of the ball. Make every motion controlled and methodical.

- Keep abdominals active.

- Lift your right knee off the ball and extend your leg behind you. Keep hips square to avoid rocking or falling.

- Come back to center and repeat on other side.

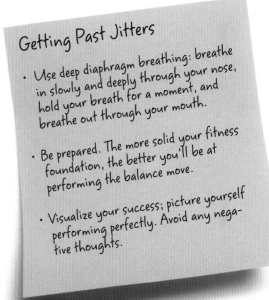

Getting Past Jitters

- Use deep diaphragm breathing: breathe in slowly and deeply through your nose, hold your breath for a moment, and breathe out through your mouth.

- Be prepared. The more solid your fitness foundation, the better you'll be at performing the balance move.

- Visualize your success; picture yourself performing perfectly. Avoid any negative thoughts.

UPPER BODY WITH BALANCE

To improve fitness and strength gains, incorporate upper-body lifting into your stability balance program

Once you have mastered the ability to kneel on a stability ball, you can incorporate upper-body strength-training moves. Functionally, this is the pinnacle of stability ball training. The combination of balance, coordination, and strength needed to engage in these exercises creates a multifaceted challenge.

How is this functional, you ask? Imagine you are on a sailboat during a storm. The boat is rocking on a choppy sea and you need to make an adjustment to the rigging. To accomplish this task, you will need to simultaneously engage your balance, core stability, and upper-body strength. Can you think of other real-life scenarios that combine balance, core

Balance Workout: Position 1

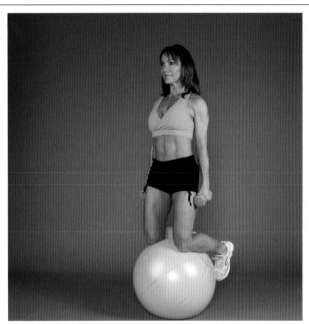

- Practice this without dumb-bells first.

- Come up into four-point ball balance position. Roll knees forward as you activate your inner-thigh muscles.

- Engage abdominals and lift upper body off the ball in one motion. Touching toes to the back of the ball helps balance.

- Keep arms at your sides, palms facing each other.

Balance Workout: Position 2

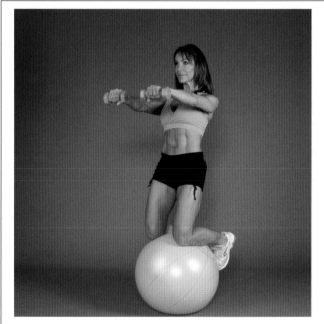

- Abdominal strength and relaxed breathing will keep you upright.

- Do not make big recovery movements. Keep righting yourself with small, subtle moves.

- With shoulders retracted, raise arms to the front of your body, palms down.

- Keep eyes focused ahead of you.

stability, and strength? How about carrying a heavy object down attic stairs? Your training will help you in all situations where you need full cooperation from your body.

You probably will not be able to lift the same amount of weight as you can when doing these exercises on a stable surface. Consequently, use these exercises as a functional variation and not as your sole upper-body strength-training program.

The importance of a quality stability ball cannot be emphasized enough. Unfortunately, not all balls are created equally; cheap balls will not hold their shape, regardless of inflation. Contrary to what you might think, these exercises are easier to perform on a firm ball than a squishy one. Quality fitness balls will support a high static load and be burst resistant; this means they will deflate slowly if accidently punctured. Therapists and trainers recommend DuraBall brand. Quality balls are a good value because they last longer. Unlike their inexpensive counterparts, reputable manufacturers provide defect guarantees and a good return policy. Make sure you select a ball size that is best for your height.

Balance Workout: Position 3

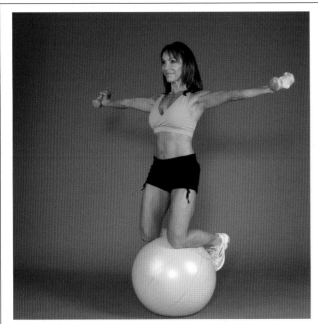

- Externally rotate your arms while they are in front of your body. With palms up, extend arms to the sides, parallel to the floor.

- Adding rotation and transferring your weight from front to sides help hold your core in place.

- Tuck your pelvis under slightly and extend your torso length.

Balance Workout: Position 4

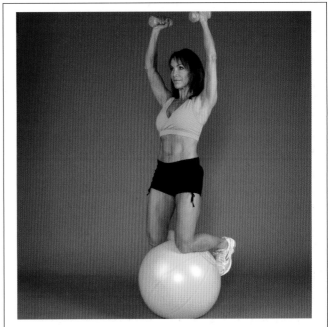

- Keep dumbbells palms up and raise them overhead.

- Do not lock your elbows.

- Internally rotate arms and bring dumbbells back down to start position at sides, palms facing each other.

- Focus on increasing your comfort level and improving proficiency rather than the number of reps or amount of weight.

GLIDER SERIES

Gliders are a functional piece of equipment to help you move smoothly, continuously, and effortlessly (almost)

The manufacturers of gliders call them a revolution. While this exercise tool may not qualify as a fundamental and transformational change to our culture, they sure are a great new functional-fitness gadget. A fitness glider is a sliding disc exercise system that transforms movements into smooth, graceful lines of flowing motion. Functionally speaking, women of all fitness levels are capable of using sliding discs in their training program.

Designed by a woman, Gliding discs are high-tech polymer discs about the size of a paper plate. There are two styles: one for use on hardwood floors and one for carpets. This makes them a great, portable, all-purpose option.

Glider Toe Stand

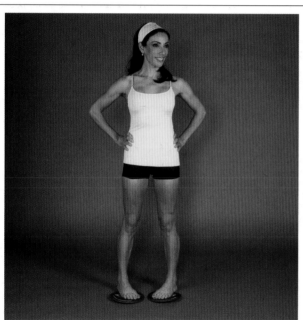

- Place balls of your feet on Gliding discs and stand in neutral body position.

- Internally rotate your toes, initiating action from your hips, not your feet.

- Lengthen inner thighs and reach your legs long. Knees should point in the same direction as the toes during movement.

- Reverse to external rotation using the same technique.

Glider Ballet Sweep

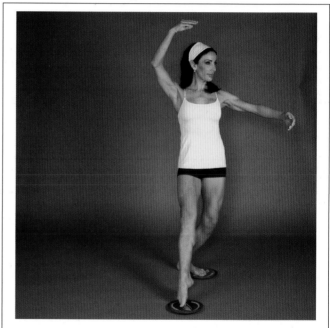

- Place your left foot and right toe on Gliding discs. Start in ballet posture with upper body lifted, shoulders retracted, and abdominals engaged.

- Sweep your right foot forward, to the right, and back behind your body in one graceful motion. rotating from the hip socket.

- Repeat with other leg.

Gliding exercises can incorporate a full range of motion or smaller movements. Sliding is a non-impact movement, meaning it is easy on the joints. The gliding motion creates a sensation of grace and beauty.

Gliding discs are akin to "training wheels" for ballet movements. In ballet, the dancer is asked to avoid bracing, tension, or excess effort. Sliding your legs across the floor simulates a dancer's seamless motion. Start off by becoming aware of the contact between your feet and the floor. Heightened awareness of weight transition minimizes strain on the body.

Glider Reverse Pike Start

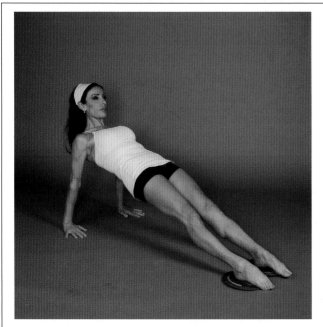

- Place heels on center of Gliding discs. Assume reverse plank position.

- Keep hips high and avoid sinking buttocks toward the floor.

- Lift chest high and actively press hands to the floor, taking pressure off your wrists.

- Keep head forward to reduce neck strain.

Glider Reverse Pike Finish

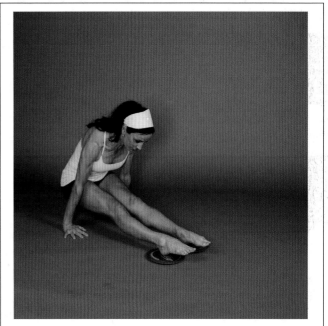

- Engage abdominals and reach the arms as long as possible.

- Soften pressure on your heels, lift buttocks slightly, and sweep hips through the arms.

- Avoid dropping buttocks to the floor. Hold pike and, if possible, lift feet off the floor.

GLIDER CRAWL

Your body should move itself around efficiently under a wide variety of circumstances

The next time you are hoisting your body up for whatever reason, or racing across the airport terminal to catch a plane, you'll be happy you prepared yourself with calisthenics. The name *calisthenics* is of Greek origin. It combines two words, *kalos,* meaning "beautiful," and *sthénos,* meaning "strength."

Calisthenics is classified as a form of physical exercise closely related to, but not part of, gymnastics. Repeating an exercise over and over, for an extended period of time, is what gives you muscular endurance. Considering gymnasts are said to be the strongest people on the planet pound for pound, training with calisthenics is validated.

The mountain climber and inchworm sculpt the abs, stretch

Glider Mountain Climber Start

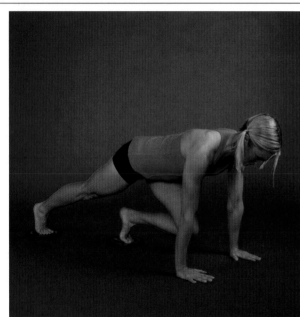

- Place Gliding discs under the balls of your feet and palms shoulder-width apart on the floor.

- Start with hips lifted in the basic push-up position.

- Bring left knee forward toward your chest without lifting your foot off the glider.

- Maintain equal pressure on both feet.

Glider Mountain Climber Finish

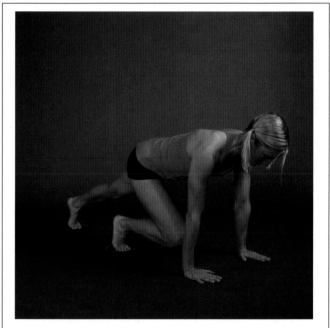

- Simultaneously return left leg back and bring right knee forward toward your chest.

- Use your abdominals to initiate the movement to lessen the focus on the hip flexors.

- Keep shoulders, chest, and hips parallel to the floor. Avoid excessive rounding of the spine.

- Variation: Knees to outside of arms.

the body, improve upper- and lower-body shape, and build endurance. For feet and leg development, it is important to train the feet and toes to point in the same direction that you are moving. This is beneficial when you are walking, running, and going up and down stairs.

The Gliding discs provide a perfect tool to perform both of these calisthenics exercises. Rotating your feet and body into proper alignment is a smooth process. Commit to perfect form when training with gliders. This will optimize the effectiveness of your body and transfer over to everyday movements.

Glider Inchworm Start

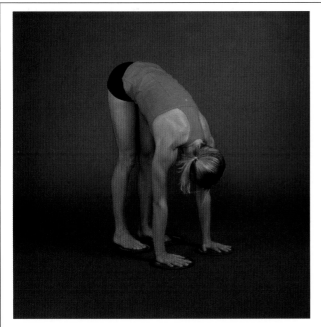

- To inchworm forward, you will need some room!

- Start with Gliding discs under your feet and your hands in a forward bend position.

- Slide your hands forward into a plank position, keeping your feet stationary.

Glider Inchworm Finish

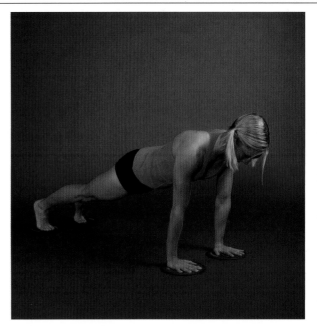

- From plank position, anchor your hands, contract abdominals, and lift hips toward the ceiling, sliding the feet toward your palms.

- Fold your body forward, bending from hips and maintaining neutral spine.

- Keep hands and feet on the floor.

WARM-UP, COOLDOWN

A cooldown will decrease your body temperature and remove waste products from the working muscles

We have already discussed how you should begin every workout with a warm-up. The warm-up increases blood circulation and prepares your muscles and heart for lifting. Conversely, the cooldown phase slows your heart rate and helps transition your body back to everyday life. The exercises below can be used both for warming up before and cooling down after the superset exercises in this chapter. Post-workout stretching promotes circulation and minimizes muscle stiffness. After a workout, your muscles are warm and pliable, which means you can get a deeper stretch and improved flexibility.

While we are talking about stretching, let's identify the different methods of stretching. Ballistic stretching uses abrupt

Ball Warm-up Start

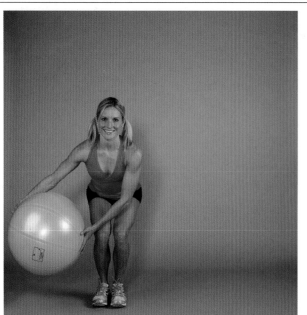

- With legs and feet together, squat to 45 degrees.

- Retract shoulders and engage abdominals. Keep torso and toes forward.

- Hold ball low to the floor on right side with both hands.

Ball Warm-up Finish

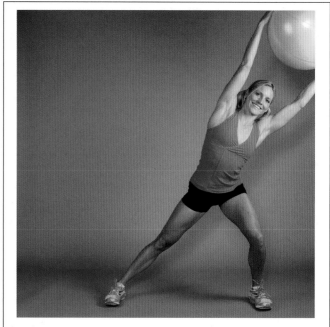

- Straighten your legs and lunge to your left, bringing the ball diagonally in front of your body until it reaches overhead to your left side.

- Use abdominals to initiate controlled diagonal wood-

- chopper movement.

- Avoid swinging the ball.

- Return to start and repeat on other side for a total of ten minutes for both sides.

movement, forcing the body past a normal range of motion via momentum. Dynamic stretching involves gradual movement, increasing the reach gently. Static stretching holds a stretch at a comfortably challenging position. Passive stretching involves outside assistance to hold the stretch. Isometric stretching requires tensing the muscles against static resistance.

Of all these methods, dynamic and static stretching are recommended. If you have the benefit of a qualified assistant, then proprioceptive neuromuscular facilitation (PNF), or post-isometric relaxation, is a great option. This method alter-

nates between an assisted passive stretch and an isometric stretch of the same muscle.

Ballistic stretching is highly discouraged. Using a bouncing movement to stretch is dangerous and increases the risk of injury. Any time you move, swing, or bounce at speed, moving a limb beyond its normal range of motion, you are working against the body's myotatic stretch reflex. Myotatic stretch reflex is a contraction of a muscle in response to stretching its tendon. Your muscle spindles inside the muscle cells are there to protect you, so do your best not to override them.

Ball Back Bend

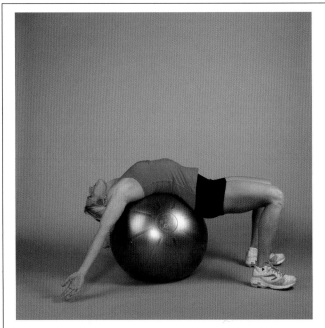

- Back bend is a cooldown and relaxation position.

- Sit on the ball and walk feet forward until your low back is centered on top. Keep your feet on the floor shoulder-width apart.

- Extend hands overhead and curl back over the ball to facilitate spinal traction.

- Allow head to hang.

Ball Forward Bend

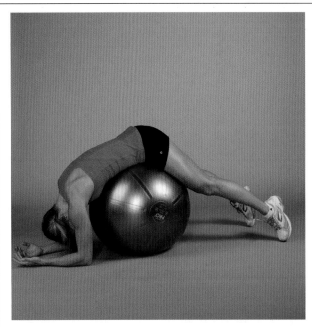

- Ball forward bend is a cooldown and relaxation position.

- Lie with belly over the ball and curl forward until hips,

chest, and upper thighs are pressing against the top.

- Allow head, arms, and feet to hang over the ball.

CORE

The word *core* means the central or inner part, the essence or most important matter

Supersets are a great choice for burning more calories and engaging more muscles in less time. They are considered an advanced method of working out. Conventional weight training uses straight sets, where you do a series of repetitions of one exercise, rest, and do another set. In a superset, you do one set of a particular exercise then perform another set of a different exercise, using a different muscle group.

Supersets increase the intensity of your training session. By doing two exercises back-to-back, you have eliminated the rest time between static sets. No rest time means a harder workout. If your program design is such that you have been doing the same routine for over eight weeks, supersets pro-

Pass the Ball: Position 1

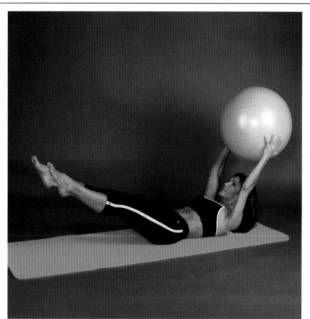

- Lie on your back with neutral body position and hold the ball between your hands overhead.

- Lift both legs and arms (with ball) off the mat at the same time, using abdomi-

nals to initiate the movement.

- Back peels off mat one vertebra at a time. Keep shoulders away from ears.

Pass the Ball: Position 2

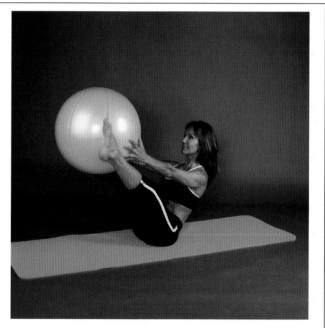

- Continue coming up to V-up position, passing the ball from extended arms to extended legs.

- Balance on your sit bones to maintain form during

transfer. Take time to position the ball well.

- Hold the ball at your ankles, but squeeze from inner thighs.

vide the variety needed to get you to the next plateau.

The time-saving advantage of supersets is obvious. Supersets are especially attractive to women, as we tend to be natural multitaskers. We multitask in so many aspects of our lives that we are already superset minded. Training different body parts, one after another, means a more efficient and productive workout, inspiring feelings of accomplishment and satisfaction.

To really take it up a notch, superset with compound exercises when performing core training. The combination is a jackpot.

Pass the Ball: Position 3

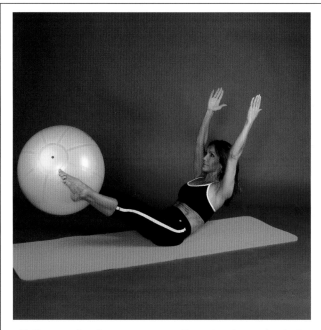

- Roll your spine down slowly, one vertebra at a time toward the mat.

- Hollow your lower abdominals by performing a vacuum, where you pull the navel to your spine.

- Do not arch your back at any point. Keep neck long and shoulders retracted.

- Attempt to continue movement without resting on the floor.

Supersetalicious

- Supersets are deliciously time efficient and effective.

- Superset training refers to doing alternating exercises back-to-back with minimal rest. Supersets may alternate agonist-antagonist muscles or different exercises using the same muscle group.

- Train your back with a set of hyperextensions between your abdominal routines for agonist-antagonist muscle group training. Do a transversus abdominis and rectus abdominis, both abdominal muscle exercises like Pass the Ball, for same muscle group training.

CHEST-BACK
Compound supersets are the most demanding and taxing on your body and nervous system

The upper-body superset is a compound superset. Considered one of the most taxing forms of superset training, it requires 100 percent of your energy and attention. It will produce results in a short amount of time. Because compound superset training is harder on the nervous system, much like stability ball functional training, post-session recovery is vital.

Supersets often alternate agonist and antagonist muscles. This means you are working a target muscle and its opposing muscle. This is achieved in our compound superset below by alternating between a stability ball chest press and a bent-over row, which works the mid-back. Similarly, a chest-fly exercise is alternated with a reverse fly for the back. The benefit

Chest Press

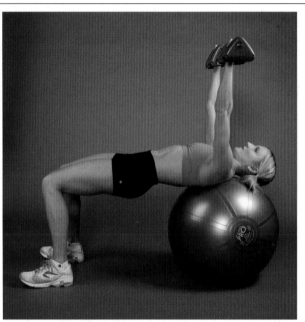

- Assume bridge position with upper back on top of the ball, feet shoulder-width apart and hips parallel to the floor.

- Perform chest press exercise with steady tempo.

- The importance of having a correctly sized stability ball is key for proper lifting form.

One-Arm Row

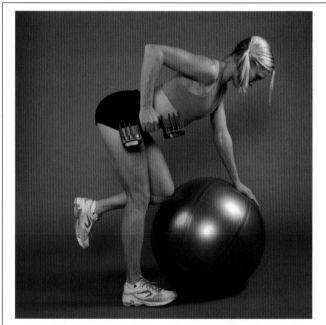

- When finished with chest exercise, position body by side of the ball in preparation for one-arm row.

- Keep your knee to the back and your hand to the front of the ball, creating an op-

positional force upon which to actively press.

- Perform one-arm row.

- Repeat with other arm.

to this form of superset training is that by switching from the chest to the back, you give one muscle group a rest while the other is being taxed. By alternating with agonist and antagonist muscles, you also maintain symmetry of strength.

If you want to walk away from your superset session shaking like a leaf and utterly spent, try alternating exercises that work the same muscle group. For example, alternate between the chest press and the chest fly.

Be aware that same muscle group compound supersets will preexhaust your muscles and you may not be able to lift an equal amount of weight on your second set. Adjust your weight or number of repetitions accordingly so that you maintain the excellent form we've been working on!

Speaking of how much weight to use, remember that there is no point to weight lifting if you don't use a meaningful amount of resistance. Always choose a weight you can lift with proper form for 12 repetitions, give or take. If by your final set you can only do 8 reps, that is fine and may often be the case when you increase the resistance or difficulty of a given exercise.

Fly

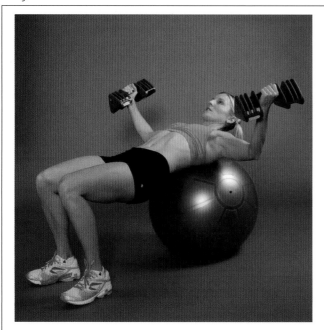

- Keeping only your mid upper back on the ball and your head unsupported creates more stability to the shoulders, but less to the neck flexors.

- Keep hips parallel to the floor and shoulders retracted.

- Perform chest fly with steady tempo, bringing dumbbells together in hugging motion.

Reverse Fly

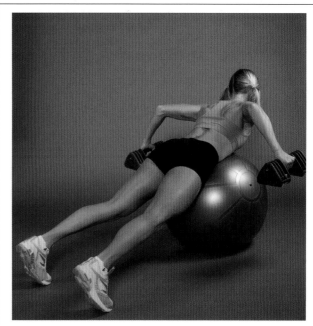

- Lie with your belly on the ball with neutral spine. Retract shoulders.

- Use light weights to focus on back posture muscles. The rear delts will work, too.

- Use same motion as front fly, only in reverse. Lift weights to shoulder level and avoid straining to pull elbows behind torso.

BICEPS-TRICEPS-SHOULDERS

In terms of productivity and intensity, supersets of three muscle groups are highly effective

There are a number of weight-training superset options. Supersets can be done by alternating three muscle groups as well. Considering we just completed a chest-back superset, this superset rounds out the upper body nicely by allowing us to combine the shoulders, biceps, and triceps.

This is also a great time-efficient way to get your shoulders in on a superset, Because the shoulders have no antagonist muscle group, it's challenging to come up with a good exercise to superset the shoulders with. By combining shoulders and arms into one triple superset, your efficiency is optimized.

By doing this triple superset using a stability ball, we have upped the ante. The biceps curl, skull crusher, and triceps kick-

Seated Biceps Curl

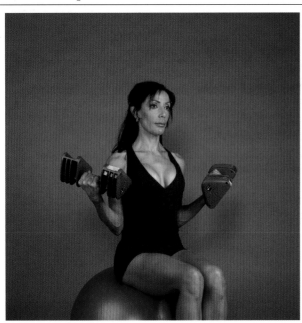

- Sit on a stability ball with neutral body position, dumbbells by your sides with palms facing each other.

- Retract shoulders and engage abdominals.

- Keep elbows tucked to the sides of your body.

- Perform biceps curls with steady tempo.

One-Arm Skull Crusher

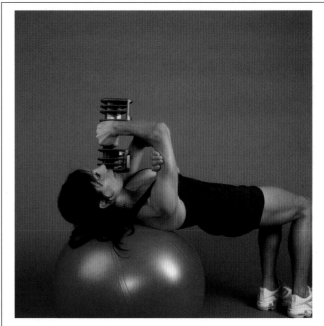

- Position upper back on top of ball in a bridge position, feet on the floor.

- Raise right arm overhead, holding the dumbbell palm in. Use left hand to stabilize the upper right arm.

- Drop lower right arm diagonally over your face until elbow comes to 90-degree angle.

- Repeat with other arm.

backs shown here are all traditionally isolation exercises. By using a stability ball instead of a bench, you add core strength and balance to the challenge. It's a triple superset delight!

Keep in mind that one shoulder exercise is not enough to thoroughly work the three muscle groups of the shoulder. However, one exercise each for the biceps and triceps in a workout session is sufficient. This is because the biceps and triceps are small muscles that fatigue easily. Don't worry: We've got a great way to work in more supersetting shoulder action a bit later in this chapter.

Seated Shoulder Press

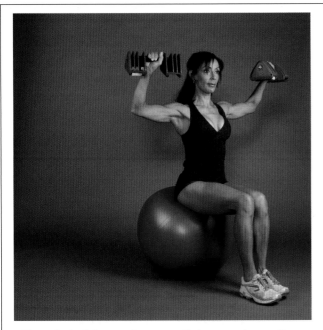

- Sit on the ball, feet on the floor.

- Retract shoulders and engage your core.

- Perform overhead press with controlled tempo.

- To keep tension on the shoulders, return upper arms so they are just parallel to the floor.

One-Arm Kickback

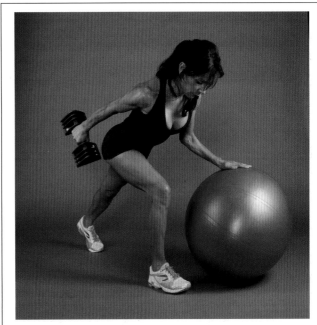

- Come into right leg forward lunge position with left hand over the top of the ball.

- Perform triceps kickbacks, focusing on straight-arm technique, which also targets the shoulders.

- Keep hips square and maintain an equal balance between both legs and left hand.

- Repeat with other arm.

QUADS-HAMSTRINGS

Once you complete a squat, do some dead lifts for a complementary, time-efficient training session

Sure, you might be strapped for time, but superset training is not just a girl-on-the-go alternative. It will provide limitless options to your workout routine, keeping your muscles guessing and you motivated. The front and back of your legs comprise another antagonistic, yin-yang superset training option.

Squats and dead lifts provide a wonderful complement to one another during a superset session. If you are working with a stability ball, use the ball as your prop for both. To help with recall, try mentally categorizing these two exercises as the two-leg and one-leg versions of quad-ham supersets.

The stability ball program will not be the same as doing

Wall Squat

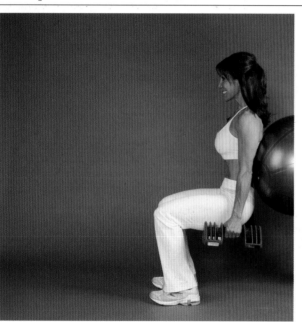

- Place the ball behind your back and against a wall. Hold dumbbells by your sides, palms facing each other.

- Maintain neutral spine and engage abdominals.

- Press weight into heels and perform wall squats, bringing upper thighs parallel to the floor. Return to standing by flexing quads and glutes.

- Avoid using momentum.

Ball Straight-Leg Dead Lift

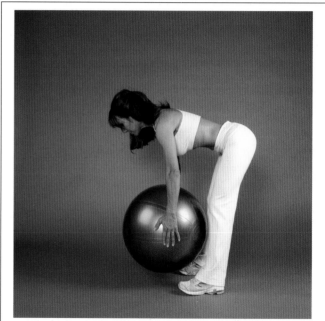

- Stand in neutral body position, feet shoulder-width apart.

- Press the ball between your hands. Retract shoulders and engage abdominals.

- Keep the ball close as you lower, hinging at the hips. Stretch the hamstrings.

- Shift hips forward, engage inner thighs, and press through heels to lift back to standing.

the exercises on a stable surface with heavier weight. For one, you won't be lifting as much weight, which means less muscle fiber recruitment, less muscle mass gains, and less calorie and fat-burning benefits.

What you will accomplish with the ball is functional training, toning, and increased balance to both sides of your legs. Placing your foot on the stability ball and performing a one-leg static squat or lunge, coupled with a hamstring one-leg curl-up, is brutal—brutal in a good way!

Change your quad-ham superset routine to one of the many exercise options listed in previous chapters. The idea is to continue performing front of the leg moves with back of the leg moves. Or, if you want to employ same muscle-group training, try a reverse lunge to a side lunge or an overhead squat to a plié squat.

Advanced Stability Lunge

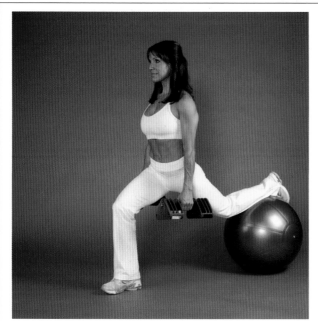

- Start in forward lunge position with right leg forward and left leg resting on top of the ball.

- With dumbbells by your sides, palms facing each other, retract shoulders and engage abdominals.

- Perform static lunges, keeping even weight between both points of contact.

- Repeat with other leg.

Leg-up Hamstring Lift

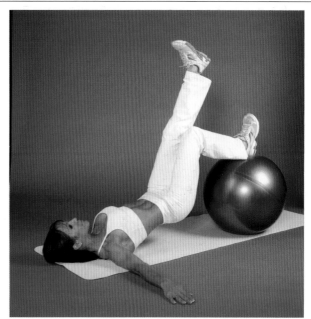

- Lie on your back and place right heel on top of the ball with left leg extended toward the ceiling.

- Press your right heel into the ball and perform leg-up lifts, keeping the ball stationary.

- Repeat lift without a full rest in between reps. Keep torso erect throughout the movement.

SHOULDERS-CALVES

Perform two exercises in a row with little rest in between for more effective training

Staggering a superset is when you exercise major muscles with minor muscles, or completely unrelated muscles. For example, you can alternate between working your shoulders and calves. The calves and shoulders are not agonist-antagonistic, but by training two completely unrelated muscles, you still get the increased intensity and time efficiency as with any superset.

This also fits perfectly with the supersets already described in this chapter. If you have used the biceps-triceps-shoulders superset discussed earlier, you can get more shoulder work in while maintaining your superset momentum. Shoulders and calves are not the only stagger superset option. Any two unrelated muscle groups can work: abs and calves, quads

Seated Lateral Side Raise

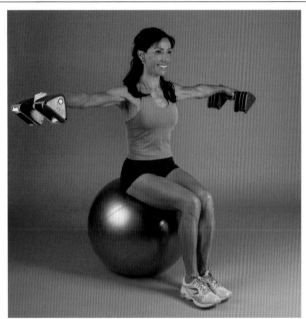

- Sit on the ball with feet on the floor.

- Perform lateral side raise with controlled tempo.

- Holding the dumbbells with the wrists slightly bent

takes pressure off forearms and transfers more work to the shoulders.

- Do not lift weights higher than your shoulders.

Donkey Calf Raise

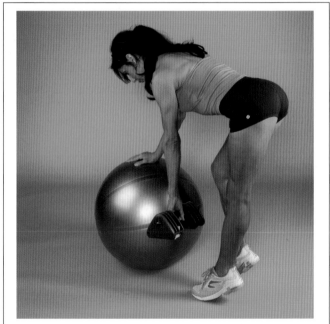

- Place right hand on the ball. Bend forward until back is parallel to the floor. Weight hangs from left hand.

- Balance on left foot and place right foot on left anklebone.

- Perform calf raises. Repeat with other leg.

- Variation: Have someone sit on your low back like a donkey ride.

and shoulders, abs and shoulders. You get the idea.

The time efficiency associated with using supersets conjures up visions of trying to squeeze in a full-body workout in a minimum amount of time. However, some people choose to divide their workouts by body parts, using intensified sessions (see chapter 18). Staggered supersets can be used in this vein to dedicate a complete training session to two separate muscle groups.

For example, if you want to focus on shoulder and abs during one workout session, you might do two or three sets each of lateral side raises, overhead presses, and rear delt exercises. In between each set, you could train your abdominals by doing stability ball crunches, bicycle obliques, and reverse crunches.

Make a note, however, that if you stagger superset training your abdominals with your upper body, you may not want to use the stability ball for the upper-body exercises. This is because any exercise on a stability ball engages your core, so you would essentially be supersetting your abdominals. Unless your objective is to completely obliterate and tax the core, it is better to superset the calves with the chest, back, or legs.

Seated Shoulder Press

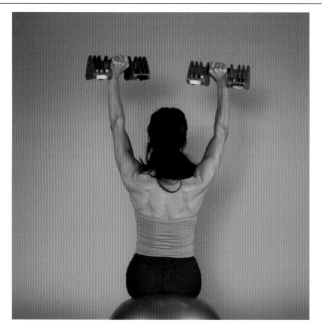

- Sit on the ball with feet on the floor. Engage abdominals to minimize stress to lower back.

- Perform overhead press.

- Concentrate on sliding

shoulders down the back, keeping space between shoulders and ears.

- Lift without locking elbows to prevent injuries and to keep stress off the shoulders.

Lying Rear Deltoid Raise

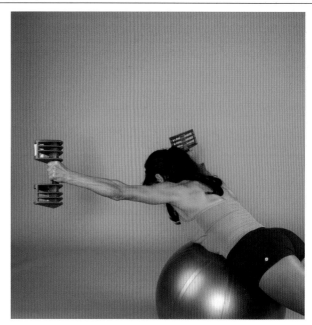

- Lie with your belly on the ball with legs extended.

- Start with dumbbells by your sides, palms facing each other.

- Raise the dumbbells to your shoulders in a semicircular motion until your biceps are parallel to the floor.

- Turn pinky side of dumbbells up and squeeze back of your shoulders.

DAY ONE

Today's session will be to train the chest, back, legs, and core

It's time to outline an eight-week, hard-core, weight-training plan that uses barbells, dumbbells, and a variety of machines. This program is intense. It is a six-day-per-week schedule, with one day off to recuperate. Each session lasts approximately one hour. The program uses a split routine, meaning you train each body part three times per week.

Always warm up before starting a session and stretch and cool down after. For focal-point exercises (noted in *italics*)

perform four or five sets of 12 to 15 reps. For all other exercises, perform two or three sets of 10 to 12 reps. For one-arm exercises, complete the same number of reps per side. Aim for ten to twenty seconds for isometrics.

Note: You won't be able to lift the same number of reps when your muscles are preexhausted. If you can only do 6 to 10 reps on later sets of a same-body-part exercise, that's perfect. Maintain correct form. If you get sloppy, decrease the weight or stop the exercise.

Flat Bench Press

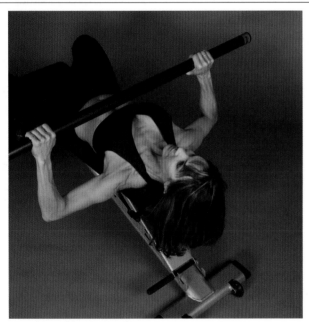

- Choose a barbell weight that allows you to lift 12 to 15 challenging reps for the first set.

- To get barbell into position, start seated with barbell on your thighs. Engage your

core and roll back onto bench with knees in fixed position so that barbell ends up over your chest.

- Perform chest press. Press head into bench to assist shoulder retraction.

One-Arm Row

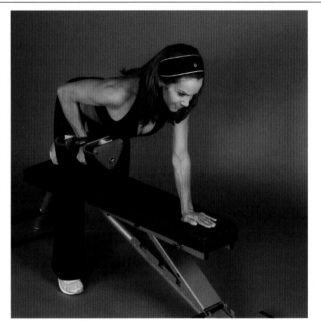

- Use grips to assist in holding heavy dumbbells (a challenging amount of weight). This allows full focus on your lats.

- Position left knee on the bench and right leg under

hip. Use left hand for support.

- Perform one-arm row, avoiding overrotating torso.

- Repeat with other arm.

208

DAY ONE EXERCISES

Superset Chest and Back
Flat Bench Press and *One-Arm Row*
Dumbbell Incline Fly and Lat Pull-Down
Wide Push-up and Seated Row

Superset Legs
Deep Barbell Squat and Dead Lift
Static Lunge and Leg-up Lift (hamstrings)

Superset Calves and Abdominals
Standing Calf Raise
Vacuum
Transversus Abdominis One-Leg Activation
Weighted Decline Crunch
Side Woodchopper

Deep Barbell Squats

- To perform a deep barbell squat, place the bar on your shoulders/upper back. Firmly grasp the bar with both hands. Descend until thighs are just past parallel to the floor.

- Execute squat with perfect neutral body position and proper alignment.

- Myth debunked: Squats are not bad for your knees or dangerous to your spine when you do them properly.

Weighted Decline Crunch

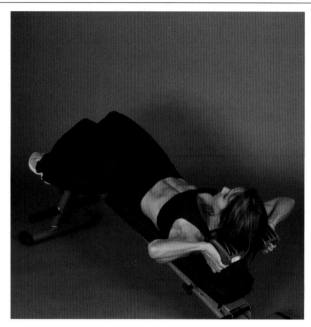

- Place feet on the bottom of a decline bench. Lie on your back and place dumbbell behind head with elbows out to the side.

- Perform decline crunches, pulling navel into spine.

- Do not rest upper back between reps.

DAY TWO

Today's session will include shoulders, arms, calves, and abdominals—plus some cardio training

Cardio training during an upper-body training day will help drop body fat and flush the system. Aim for twenty to sixty minutes of moderate-intensity cardio. This may include a brisk walk, a jog, or non-impact activities like cycling, swimming, and elliptical training. If your heart rate is so high that you can't have a conversation, you are pushing too hard. If at any point during the eight-week transformation you feel stressed and overworked, back off, or take an extra rest day.

Remember to always warm up before a session and stretch and cool down after. Follow the number of reps outlined in Day One.

Incline Overhead Press

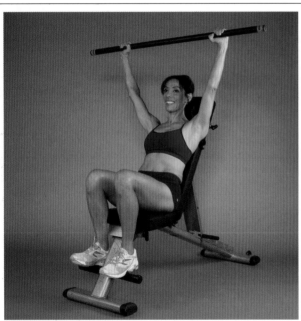

- Adjust bench to 60-degree angle. With wide grip, palms down, bring barbell above your shoulders.

- Press head into the bench, helping to lift and retract shoulders.

- Plant feet on the floor or foot-bar.

- Perform incline press, lowering bar to just above chest.

Standing Barbell Curl

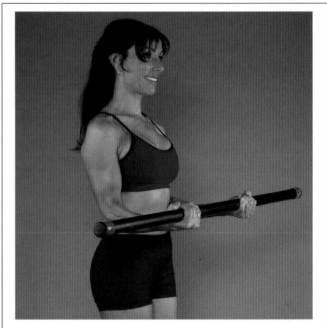

- Stand in neutral body position and grasp a barbell with palms up, shoulder-width grip.

- Retract shoulders and engage abdominals. Tuck elbows to sides of your body.

- Perform barbell curl, lifting in a wide arc from thighs to shoulder level.

- Variation: Narrow grip for more biceps.

Cardio Training (twenty to sixty minutes)

Superset Shoulders

Internal/External Rotation; *Incline Overhead Press* and Incline Dumbbell Lateral Side Raise; Upright Row and Standing Bent-over Fly

Superset Biceps and Triceps

Standing Barbell Curl and *Lying Triceps Barbell Extension,* Concentration Curl and One-Arm Kickback; Reverse Wrist Curl and Narrow Push-up

Superset Calves and Abdominals

Toes In Calf Raise; Toes Out Calf Raise; Vacuum; Transversus Abdominis One-Leg Activation; Bent Knee Raise; *Flat-Bench Flutter Kick;* Side Plank Crunch

Lying Triceps Barbell Extension

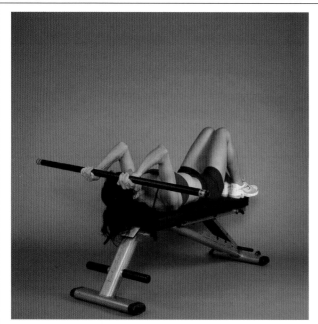

- Lie on your back using flat bench with knees bent, feet flat, shoulders retracted, and abdominals engaged.

- Hold the bar over your chest with narrow grip, palms forward, arms extended.

- Keep upper arms still, bend elbows, and lower bar overhead to a 90-degree angle.

Flat-Bench Flutter Kick

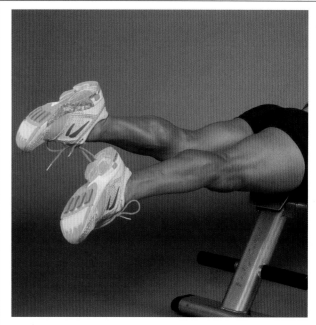

- Lie on your belly on a flat bench with hips on edge and legs extended off the back.

- Start with legs level with hips.

- Lift one leg higher than the other and alternate. Mimic the movement of a flutter kick in the water.

- Variation: Do flutter kicks while lying on your back for abdominal work.

DAY THREE

Feeling good? Time to train the chest, back, legs, and core again

The goal of weight training is to cause your muscles to adapt to the challenges presented. Intense training causes microtearing of muscle tissue. This may leave you feeling sore. The official name for this is *delayed-onset muscle soreness*. It is a necessary process for the growth of your muscles. Some people enjoy a bit of post-workout soreness, because it represents progress! If you are sore from yesterday's workout, it is not due to lactic acid build-up.

Remember to always warm up before a session and stretch and cool down after. Stay focused during your session. Once your mind starts drifting elsewhere, the quality of your training diminishes. Keep your attention on your working muscles, not on the weight you are lifting. This improves form, performance, and results.

Flat-Bench Dumbbell Fly

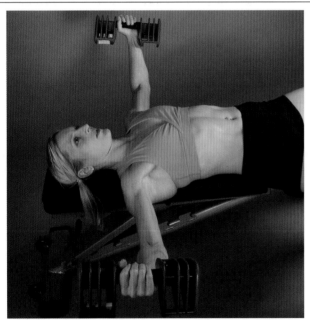

- Lie on your back. Hold dumbbells over your chest, palms facing each other. Retract shoulders and engage abdominals.

- Perform dumbbell fly, lowering dumbbells with arms fixed in a slightly bent position. Keep shoulders internally rotated.

- Concentrate on squeezing the cleavage at the top of the movement and stretching the chest at the bottom.

Flat-Bench Prone Dumbbell Row

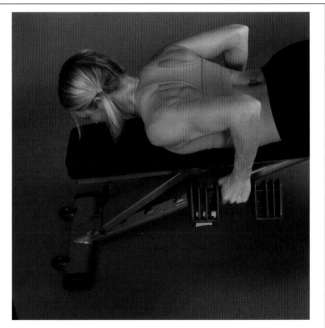

- Lie with belly down on a high bench. Tuck pelvis slightly and press thighs into the bench.

- Start with dumbbells hanging to the sides of the bench, palms facing each other.

- Retract shoulders and engage abdominals. Perform dumbbell row.

- Variations: One arm. Alternate arms.

DAY THREE EXERCISES

Superset Chest and Back

Flat-Bench Dumbbell Fly and *Flat-Bench Prone Dumbbell Row*; Incline Bench Press and One-Arm Pull-Down; Cable Crossover and Bow and Arrow; Hi-Low Push-up

Leg Training—Straight Sets and Supersets

VMO Squat; Plié Squat; Hamstring Leg Curl; *Barbell Reverse Lunge*; One-Leg Dead Lift and Walking Lunge

Superset Calves and Abdominals

One-Leg Calf Raise; Vacuum; Transversus Abdominis One-Leg Activation; Bicycle Abs; Bench *Reverse Hyperextension*

Barbell Reverse Lunge

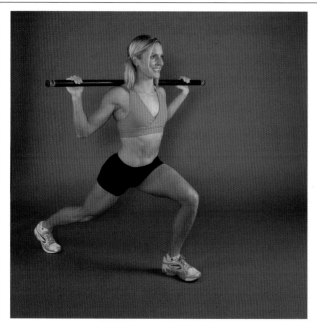

- Position barbell over upper back and hold firmly with palms forward.

- Start with feet and legs together, neutral body position. Engage abdominals.

- Perform a reverse lunge with your right leg. Repeat set with your left leg.

- Variation: Alternate legs each rep.

Bench Reverse Hyperextension

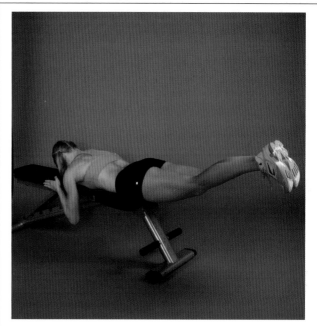

- Lie with belly on a flat bench, hips on edge, legs extended, and toes placed lightly on the floor. Hold the sides of the bench.

- Tuck pelvis under slightly and engage abdominals.

- Contract the glutes and hamstrings to lift legs level or slightly higher than hips.

- Lower to start. Move with control.

DAY FOUR

Training shoulders, arms, calves, and abdominals, combined with cardio, will fire up your metabolism

Committing to eight weeks of a rigorous schedule will improve your discipline and dramatically change your body and muscles. Keep challenging yourself.

Feel free to swap exercises for ones that work better for you. If you do alter the exercises, remember to include all the muscle-group categories: chest, back, shoulders, arms, thighs, buttocks, waist, and calves.

Always warm up before a session and stretch and cool down after. Follow the number of reps outlined in Day One.

Standing Body Bar Handoff

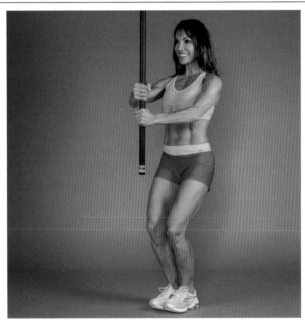

- Stand in neutral body position with knees slightly bent.

- Hold Body Bar vertically with hand low on bar.

- Retract shoulders, engage abdominals, and extend arms to front of your body.

- Walk hands up and down the bar. Do not move the bar from frontal plane.

Incline Dumbbell Biceps Curl

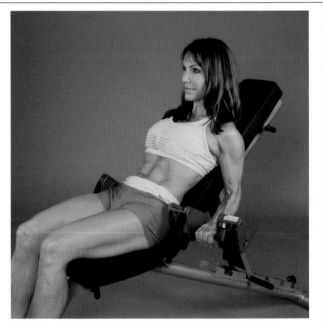

- Sit back on a 60-degree incline bench with dumbbells hanging straight by your sides, palms facing each other.

- Tuck elbows to sides of your body, externally rotating your forearms while curling the dumbbells toward your shoulders, culminating in a palms-up grip.

- Variation: Alternate arms.

DAY FOUR EXERCISES

Cardio Training (twenty to sixty minutes)

Straight Set Shoulders
Internal/External Rotation; Standing Shoulder Press; *Standing Body Bar Handoff*; Arm Circle; Seated Bent-over Fly

Superset Biceps and Triceps
Incline Dumbbell Biceps Curl and *Lying Barbell Triceps Press*; Standing Hammer Curl and Two-Arm Triceps; Kickback; Lying Curl and One-Arm Overhead Extension

Superset Calves and Abdominals
Donkey Calf Raise; Vacuum; Transversus Abdominis One-Leg Activation; *Seated Leg Tuck*; Oblique Crunch

Lying Barbell Triceps Press

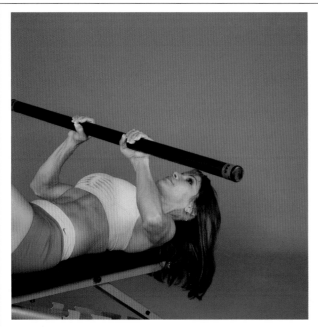

- Lie back on a flat bench with knees bent, feet flat. Retract shoulders and engage abdominals.

- Position bar over your chest with narrow, palms-down grip.

- Keep elbows tucked in and lower bar to your chest. Press back to start position.

- Do not allow elbows to point away from the sides of your body.

Seated Leg Tuck

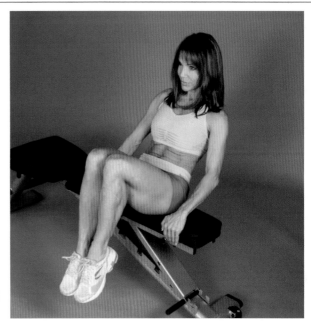

- Sit on the edge of a flat bench and grab bench on either side of your body.

- Lean back on your sit bones. Lift legs, pressing feet and legs together.

- Continue pulling legs toward your chest while crunching upper body toward your knees.

- Extend body back out while keeping tension on abdominals.

215

DAY FIVE
Have faith in the process; it's chest, back, legs, and core day once more

Reshaping your body only comes through hard work and dedication. Stick to the plan, even if sometimes you want to quit!

After the eight-week program, feel free to start mixing it up again. It will remain an important part of your body-shaping plan to make changes every six to eight weeks. Hiring a personal trainer or finding a good lifting partner is a great idea.

Keep things fresh, interesting, and challenging.

Always warm up before a session and stretch and cool down after. Follow the number of reps outlined in Day One.

This is a heavy low-back training day. Please be aware that you may need to decrease the number of sets or reps for this workout, initially.

Decline Bench Press

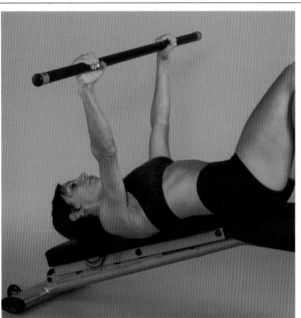

- Secure feet to the bottom of a decline bench and lie on your back.

- Hold barbell at shoulder width with palms forward. Extend arms over your chest.

- Perform decline chest press to target your lower chest and triceps.

- Modification: Consider a spotter to assist if using heavy weight.

Barbell Standing Bent-over Row

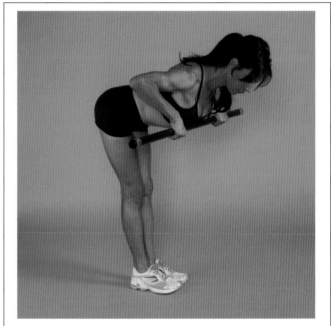

- Stand in neutral body position with barbell in front of your thighs, palms down.

- Retract shoulders and engage abdominals. Bend forward and allow barbell

- to hang vertically. Bend knees slightly.

- Maintain neutral spine and pull bar to chest, keeping elbows out to sides of the body.

DAY FIVE EXERCISES

Chest and Back—Straight Sets and Supersets
Decline Bench Press
Barbell Standing Bent-over Row
Straight-Arm Pull-over and Good Mornings
Incline Push-up

Superset Leg Training
Barbell Bench Step-up and One-Leg Squat

Reverse Plank and Stability Flex Lunge

Superset Calves and Abdominals
Reverse Calf Raise
Vacuum
Transversus Abdominis One-Leg Activation
Seated Twist
Crunches

Barbell Bench Step-ups

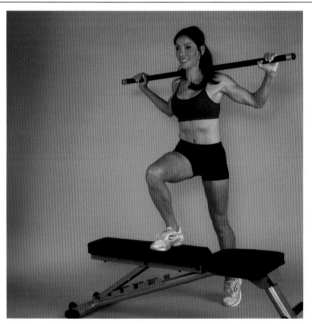

- Position barbell over your upper back and hold firmly with palms forward.

- Start with feet and legs together, neutral body position. Engage abdominals.

- Perform step-ups.

- Variations: Same leg, multiple sets. Alternate legs per rep.

Seated Twist

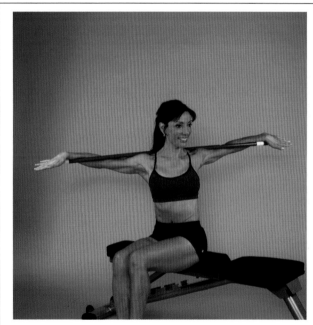

- Use a broom handle for this exercise.

- Sit on the edge of a bench with legs together, feet flat on the floor. Retract shoulders and engage abdominals.

- Keep your head and pelvis stationary and rotate upper body and shoulders as far left as possible.

- Repeat on the other side.

DAY SIX

Give today your all; do your best cardio, shoulder, arm, calf, and abdominal training yet

Keep a journal of your weekly training plan and daily progress. Make a note of the exercises performed, how many repetitions, the weight used, minutes between sets, and perceived intensity level. Start each session with a goal. At the end of the week, outline your objectives for the following week. Training logs are available online. Online companies also offer a diet tracker that keeps you on task for calories, if that is a concern.

Always warm up before a session and stretch and cool down after. Follow number of reps outlined in Day One.

Incline Rear Delt Raise

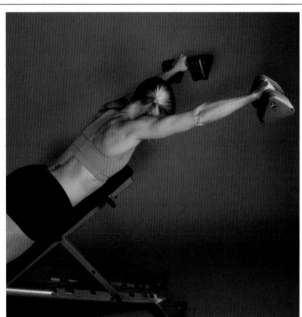

- Lie belly down on an incline bench positioned at a 45-degree angle with head extended over top of the bench.

- Start with dumbbells by your sides, palms facing each other.

- Raise dumbbells overhead in semicircular motion, ending with palms down. Do not lock elbows.

- Lower back to start position.

Inverted Reverse Grip Pull-up

- Position Body Bar between two sturdy chairs.

- Lie on the floor under the bar and hold it at shoulder width with palms facing you.

- Press heels into the floor, tighten your body, engage abdominals, and retract shoulders.

- Lift upper body using your lats until your chest touches the bar.

Cardio Training (twenty to sixty minutes)

Superset Shoulders

Internal/External Rotation; Seated Dumbbell Shoulder Press; *Incline Rear Delt Raise* (dumbbell); Low Cable Crossover and Decline Push-up

Superset Biceps and Triceps

Inverted Reverse Grip Pull-up; One-Arm Triceps Kickback;

Preacher Curl and Two-Arm Extension; Bench Dips

Superset Calves and Abdominals

Calf Raise; Reverse Calf Raise (optional); Vacuum; Transversus Abdominis One-Leg Activation; Straight-Leg Side Crunch; *Flat-Bench Leg Scissors;* V-up or One-Leg Teaser (optional)

One-Arm Triceps Kickback

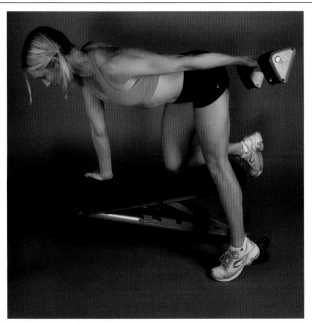

- Stand next to a flat bench with a dumbbell. Place your right knee on the bench, keep left leg straight, and use right hand for support.

- Bend left arm, bringing elbow to your side.

- Keep elbow in place and push dumbbell back and up by extending your left arm.

Flat-Bench Leg Scissors

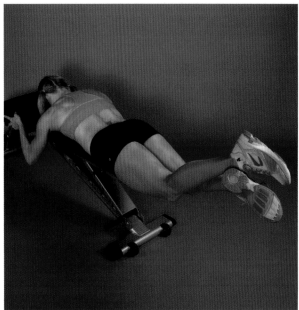

- Lie belly down on a flat bench, hips at edge. Grab the sides of the bench and rest forehead on a pad.

- Squeeze buttocks and lift legs out to sides with toes pointed.

- Alternate an over-and-under action with feet.

- Variation: Straight-leg lying scissors kick while lying on back for abdominal work.

STRETCH

Creating a daily stretching routine is easier if you schedule time on your calendar

Earlier in this book goals were addressed, along with the importance of writing them down, visualizing them, and believing that accomplishing them is possible. It is not adequate to say, "I need to stretch more every day." You must put a well thought-out plan into place.

Use your daily calendar, a palm device, or daily "to-do" list to schedule stretching and exercise. Sitting in front of the television seems like a poor alternative for a good yoga mat, but it may be just the location you need to complete your scheduled flexibility work. Stretch while standing in lines, while waiting for water to boil, and while brushing your teeth if you need to sneak in a missed session. There is no reason

Rejuvenate Reach

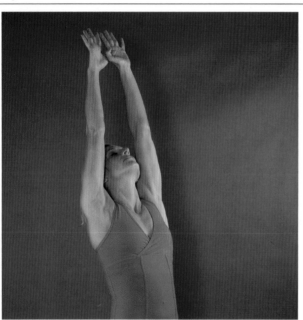

- Elongates the torso and stretches the shoulders, hands, and neck.

- Standing straight up, lace your fingers together and open up your palms.

- Extend arms and keep shoulders down. Tuck tailbone to stretch front and back of torso.

- Gently look up and lift the chin.

Roll-down Stretch

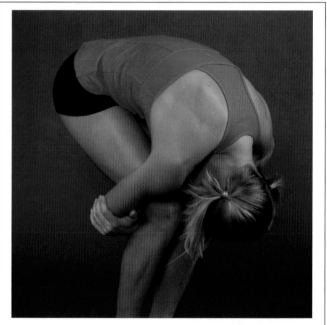

- Stretches the spine and reduces tension.

- Stand with knees slightly bent. Draw in abdominals.

- Move chin toward chest and roll torso down one vertebra at a time as far as comfortable. Keep weight centered between the feet.

- Modifications: Stand with back to a wall, or sit on the edge of a chair and roll down.

why many daily moves cannot take thirty to sixty seconds more of your time, while you hold a good stretch.

As you age, your muscles tighten and your ability to move freely and enjoy an active lifestyle may be threatened. Stretching improves mobility, reduces aches and pains, and helps coordination. It also reduces muscle tension, improves blood flow and circulation, and increases energy levels.

If that isn't the nudge you need, how about this: Stretching feels good. It's not just for pre- and post-workout training. It's an everyday, anytime addition to your well-being.

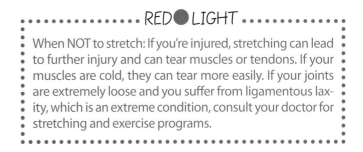
Lying Twist

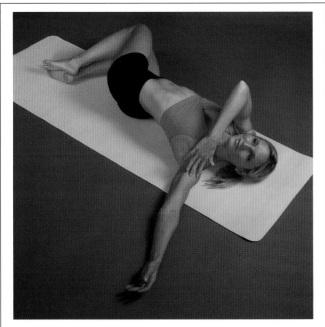

- This gently stretches the spine.

- Lie on your back; stretch arms to left.

- With knees and ankles together, roll to right side.

- Keep shoulders firmly on the mat.

- Create length between your left lower rib and hip. Turn head to look left.

Take a Bow

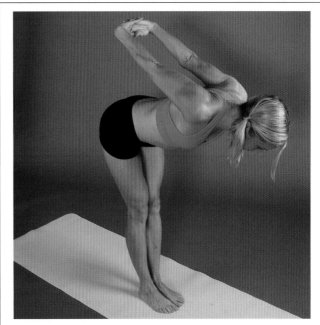

- Stretches chest and shoulders with a forward bend for the hamstrings.

- Stand with head up and shoulders retracted. Hold your hands behind the back, elbows straight.

- Raise your arms and lean forward from the hips.

- Keep back straight as you lean over.

VACUUM-CORE-FLEX

The secret to having a flat stomach is learning to vacuum and doing it daily

If you walk away with one lasting memory from this book, let it be the profound knowledge that you have a transversus abdominis (TVA) muscle. The TVA, along with the lumbar multifidus (a deep little muscle that supports your spine), is rarely mentioned in core training, yet these muscles are your "core." These muscle dynamos are your means to attaining a flat stomach and smaller midsection.

The vacuum exercise, or abdominal hollowing, is the most direct method for working inner-abdominal muscles. Once you grasp the impact the TVA muscle has on your life, neglecting it will not be an option. So, scoop and flex your abdominals daily.

Kneeling Vacuum

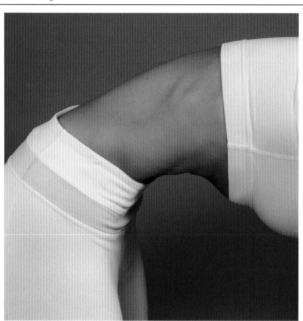

- This is a side view of hand and knees abdominal hollowing.

- To execute, completely exhale the air from your lungs.

- Suck in your stomach, pulling navel toward spine while continuing to expel air.

- Hold for ten seconds. Keep your spine still and inhale.

Core Musculature

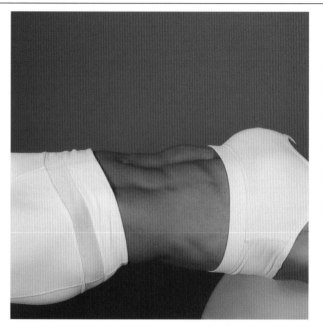

- The core includes all the muscles in the trunk.

- Build strength and endurance from the inside out.

- A weak core will not provide enough stability for efficient movements and can lead to injury.

- Enhanced functional strength and stability improve daily activity and athletic performance.

Flexing the rest of your body has benefits, too. Women who dance and practice Pilates use flexing to create lithe, strong-looking muscles. Flexing helps make the muscles hard and well defined. Blood flow to the muscles improves from squeezing and contracting.

Flexing allows you to visualize the muscle and how it's shaped. Study your body while flexing so that you can see the peak of the muscles. You'll quickly notice good points and be able to correct imbalances. With all the work you've done to create this fully functional body of yours, you owe it to yourself to flex.

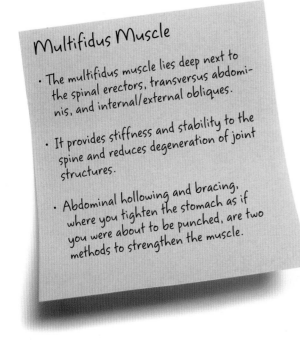

Multifidus Muscle

- The multifidus muscle lies deep next to the spinal erectors, transversus abdominis, and internal/external obliques.

- It provides stiffness and stability to the spine and reduces degeneration of joint structures.

- Abdominal hollowing and bracing, where you tighten the stomach as if you were about to be punched, are two methods to strengthen the muscle.

Biceps Flex

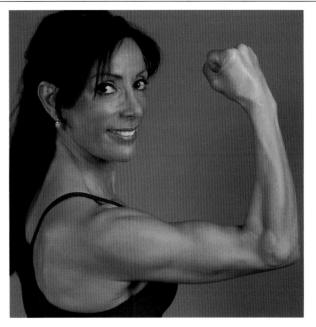

- Building beautiful arms is a goal for most women, not just for musclemen!

- Learn to flex and tighten all your muscles.

- A hard flex may cramp the muscle initially. Practice will reduce this occurrence.

DAILY MUST-DOS

223

PUSH-PULL-HANG

Your house is filled with strength-training props; use them to enhance your fitness

The items in your house are great resources for maintaining fitness. Focus on making every push and pull an opportunity to train your muscles. In a lifetime how many times will you reach overhead for a glass? How often will you pull the clothes out of the washer? How many chairs will you sit down in? How many stairs will you climb and descend?

Functional training is designed to prepare you for these everyday tasks. It's up to you to perform them with precision, attention, and deliberation. Spending hours lifting weights, practicing yoga and Pilates, and balancing on a stability ball has less value if you leave the lessons learned elsewhere.

Chairs aren't just for sitting! Try a few push-ups, using the

KNACK WEIGHT TRAINING FOR WOMEN

Chair Push-up

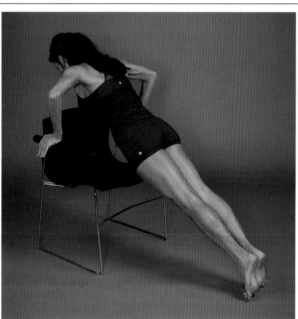

- This is essentially an incline push-up. You can also perform this on a countertop.

- Choose a sturdy chair. Place your hands flat on the arms, about shoulder-width apart.

- With legs extended behind you, lower your upper body to the chair by bending your elbows.

- Keep your body rigid.

Chair Pike

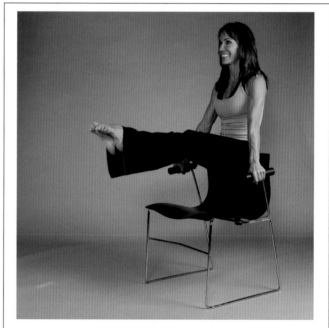

- This is a fun way to test your body-weight strength and balance.

- Sit on a chair with feet flat on the floor, hands on the arms, and elbows bent.

- Slowly press up and straighten your elbows so your bottom comes off the chair.

- Raise your legs. Aim for an L shape.

arms of the chair. Why not try a pike position, which tests your core and total body strength?

Whenever you pull something toward you, like that bag of groceries from the car, engage your abs, keep your back neutral, and use correct form.

As far as hanging is involved, do whatever it takes to find someplace sturdy to practice this amazing body-weight exercise. But please avoid hanging from bathroom towel racks, clothes hangers, and shower curtain rods.

Pulling

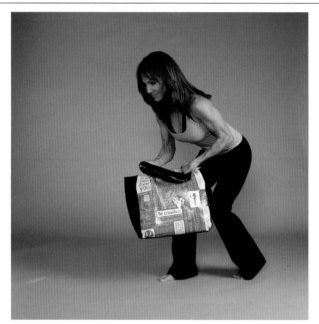

- Don't pull a fast one!

- Pulling is part of everyday activities.

- To avoid "pulling" a muscle, don't strain or overstretch.

- Use body weight and legs to help pull when you can. Make sure to engage your core so that your body is pulling as a unit, instead of getting pulled apart.

Bar Hang

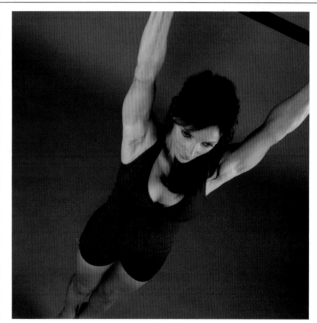

- Rock climbers use hanging to improve their static hold.

- Attempt to hang until your arms cannot hold any longer. Shake them out, wait five minutes, hang again.

- Once endurance is achieved, attempt to hang with one arm.

STEP-SQUAT-LUNGE

Keeping a toned lower body is easier once you realize that every step counts

Pedometers are great for tracking how many steps you take each day. They are technical devices that attach to your shoe, belt, wrist, or upper arm. Basic models calculate distance and calories burned; others come with health-management software to help you keep track of your fitness goals.

How many steps should you take? The precise number de-

pends. Pedometer manufacturers and walking clubs recommend 10,000 per day for active adults. Chances are, if you are taking less than 5,000 steps per day, you are living a sedentary lifestyle. Anything between 5,000 and 10,000 steps and you're on the low-to-moderate scale, and everything over 12,500 steps is highly active.

Daily Steps

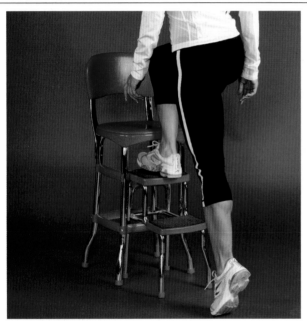

- Use a pedometer to track how many steps per day you take.

- Set a distance depending on your goals.

- Four thousand to six thousand steps are appropriate for weight loss and should incorporate uninterrupted walking.

- Consider hiking poles if training outdoors on trails.

Squat and Lift

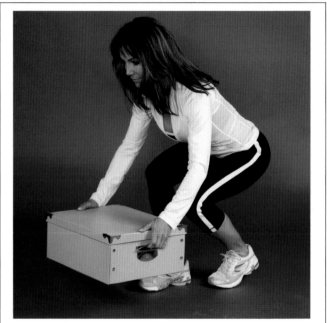

- When lifting, hold the item close to your body, as this is the strongest and most stable position.

- Bend knees and keep the back straight (neutral). Avoid twisting or bending.

- Engage abdominals and lift with your legs, keeping your eyes focused forward.

- Get help if you're straining.

Increasing your daily step quantity is easy. Try using the stairs instead of the elevator, parking farther away from your destination, or losing the car altogether!

The quality of your step, squat, and lunge is equally as important as your quantity. Practice good form to improve fitness and decrease injury. The more fit you become, the easier it will be to appreciate being able to squat down and pick things up. Performing daily tasks will have a new sense of purpose. Being "able" is good for your health.

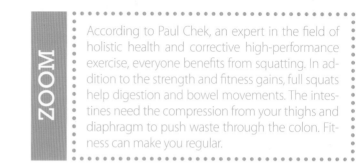
Giant Lunge

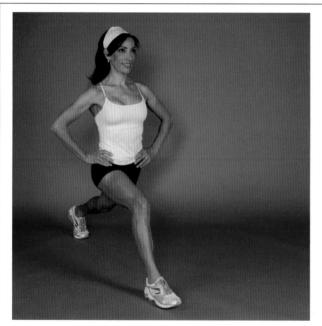

- This will firm up the upper thighs and buttocks. As always, maintain proper form.

- Start in a standing position with feet shoulder-width apart.

- Take a giant lunge forward with right foot, bending left knee until it almost, but not quite, touches the floor.

- Push off with left foot, bringing it forward into another giant lunge.

Chair Squat

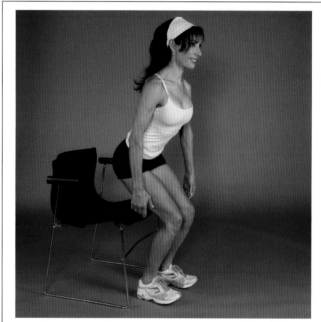

- Everytime you sit you can practice squatting! Make it a workout by not simply flopping down.

- Stand with your back toward the chair and feet shoulder-width apart. Keep head up, assume neutral spine.

- Sit down, lowering your body until legs are at a 90-degree angle.

- Contract your abdominals and quadriceps.

DAILY MUST-DOS

LISTEN-RELAX-SMILE

Stress hormones suppress the immune system; relaxation allows the body to recover and function effectively

Optimal health is a combination of physical health, spiritual wellness, and psychological, mental, and emotional well-being. Wellness includes your social network of friends, close personal relationships, career, and family (not necessarily in that order). When these factors work in harmony, chances are you are at the peak of your existence.

To *live with no regrets* is to capitalize on all that is before you. Listen to your body: What does it say? What does it need? Pause for a moment during the day and check in with your heart.

Stress causes imbalance on many levels. It opens the door to unwanted conditions and disease. In order to manage stress, you need to establish relaxation techniques. Activi-

Hear Your Heart

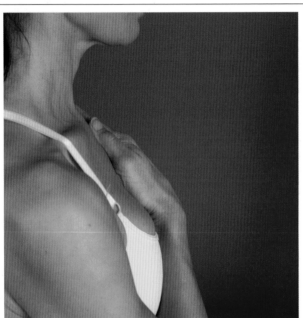

- Your heart is a muscle. If you want it to be strong, you need to exercise it.

- Please don't smoke. It can damage your heart and blood vessels.

- Eat a variety of healthy foods and avoid foods high in unhealthy fats.

Relax

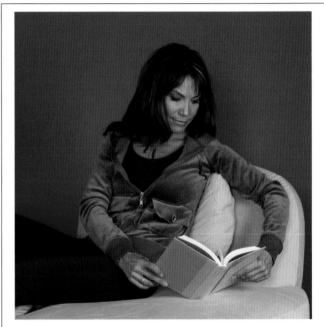

- Relaxation training has been shown to lessen or alleviate disease and conditions, including chronic and severe pain.

- Deep relaxation decreases activity of the sympathetic nervous system.

- Books provide a world of escapism and adventure, helping relieve stress.

ties that have been shown to effectively break the train of everyday thoughts and consequently calm the stress-related activity of the sympathetic nervous system include meditation, yoga, biofeedback, progressive muscle relaxation, and repetitive prayer. To master these techniques takes dedication and further research on your part.

Changes do not happen overnight. It took years to get where you are now. One step at a time will get you where you want to go. Be kind to yourself and realize that nobody's perfect. Any lapse you may have is just a temporary setback.

········· GREEN ● LIGHT ··············

Stay on course. When it comes to fitness, you need aerobic activity, strength training, and flexibility to maximize results. Commit to optimum health and wellness by practicing good habits and balance. Ultimately remember that *you* are responsible for *you*.

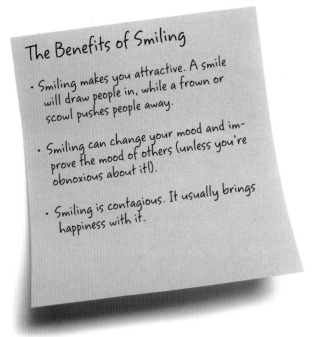

The Benefits of Smiling

• Smiling makes you attractive. A smile will draw people in, while a frown or scowl pushes people away.

• Smiling can change your mood and improve the mood of others (unless you're obnoxious about it!).

• Smiling is contagious. It usually brings happiness with it.

Smile

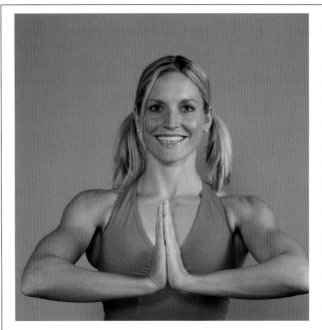

• Smiling is a form of stress release and boosts your immune system.

• It releases endorphins, serotonin, and other natural painkillers responsible for feeling good.

• Smiling improves the muscles in your face, helping you appear younger.

DAILY MUST-DOS

229

RESOURCES

The health and fitness industry has an abundant selection of resources. The Web is ripe with information, products, and services. The resources listed here point you in the right direction for exceptional accessories, assistance, and must-have home equipment. You will quickly discover that many sites offer a variety of the same equipment. To eliminate frustration, use the specific product manufacturer listed for the equipment and references used in this book.

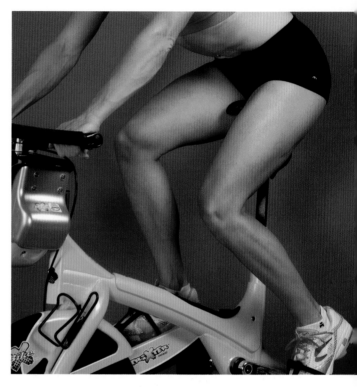

Equipment

Accu-Measure Body Fat Calipers www.accumeasurefitness.com
Adjustable Dumbbells by SelectaBell www.thecontour.com
Bench www.bodysolid.com
Body Bars www.bodybar.com
Bosu www.bosu.com
Clothing
  Running/Cycling/Fitness www.skirtsports.com
  Outdoor www.patagonia.com
  Yoga/Pilates www.lululemon.com
Cycling Shoes and Accessories
  www.shimano.com
  www.pearlizumi.com
Duraball Stability Ball www.duraball.com
E-Stim Abs www.thecontour.com
Elastic Toners www.oxygenfit.com
Elliptical Trainers
  www.lifefitness.com
  www.precor.com
Free Motion Cable System www.freemotionfitness.com
Gliders www.glidingdiscs.com
Heart Rate Monitor www.polar.com, www.nike.com
Home Gyms www.bowflex.com
Indoor Cycling Bike www.x-biking.com
Kettlebells www.kettlebellconcepts.com
Log Journal (free) www.thecontour.com
Medicine Balls www.power-systems.com

Nautilus www.nautilus.com
Outdoor Road and Mountain Bikes
  www.trek.com
  www.giant.com
  www.marinbikes.com
  www.santacruzmtb.com
Pedometers www.REI.com
Power Grips www.versagripps.com
Push-up Handles www.perfectpushup.com
Running Shoes www.newtonrunning.com
Socks www.wigwam.com
Stability Disc www.power-systems.com
Stackable Steps www.performbetter.com

Sunglasses www.oakley.com
Tanita Bioelectric Impedance Analysis Scale
 www.tanita.com
Treadmills
 www.lifefitness.com
 www.precor.com
 www.reebokfitness.com
Wobble Boards www.performbetter.com
Yoga Mat and Products
 www.lululemon.com
 www.manduka.com

Home Shopping
Home Shopping Network www.hsn.com
QVC www.qvc.com

Nationwide Fitness Facilities
24 Hour Fitness www.24hourfitness.com
Bally Total Fitness www.ballyfitness.com
Gold's Gym www.goldsgym.com
Lifetime Fitness www.lifetimefitness.com
YMCA www.ymca.net

Services
Athletic Training www.trainright.com
Bike Skills, Clinics, and Adventures
 www.bikeskills.com
 www.jimenacycling.com
 www.westernspirit.com
 www.vailmountainbikecamps.com
Boulder Center for Sports Medicine
 www.bch.org
Calorie Counter www.caloriesperhour.com
Cycling Clubs www.usacycling.com

Massage Therapy www.massagetherapy.com
Mountain Bike Organization www.imba.com
Naturally Caffeinated
 www.naturallycaffeinated.com
Personal Training
 www.ideafit.com
 www.activemary.com
 www.chekinstitute.com
Pilates Training www.pilates.com
Running Groups www.rrca.org
Support Groups www.dailystrength.com
Weight Management www.mayoclinic.com
Yoga Classes www.yogajournal.com

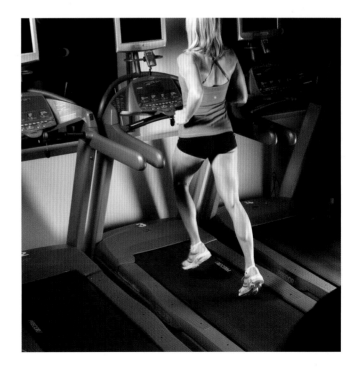

GLOSSARY

Abduction Moving away from the centerline of the body.

Abs Rectus abdominis muscles.

Accu-Measure Body Fat Calipers Personal body fat tester. The device measures fat accurately, privately, consistently, and easily.

Adduction Moving toward the centerline of the body.

Adjustable bench A weight bench that can be positioned in various ways to increase the variety of exercises that can be done on it.

Aerobic exercise Also called cardiovascular training (cardio), aerobic exercise conditions the heart and respiratory system. Cardio increases your capacity to work, burns fat, and helps keep fat off your body.

Agonist A muscle that causes specific movement via its own contraction. Agonists are also referred to as prime movers because they are primarily responsible for generating a specific movement.

Antagonist A muscle that acts in opposition to the specific movement generated by the agonist and is responsible for returning a limb to its initial position. Antagonistic muscles are found in pairs called antagonistic pairs. These consist of an extensor muscle, which opens the joint, and a flexor muscle, which does the opposite.

Anterior To the front; for example, the anterior deltoid is on the front of your shoulder.

Barbell A bar to which weights are attached at each end.

Bench Equipment resembling a park bench and used as a platform for performing weight training. Adjustable benches allow you to configure the height and angle, providing a variety of exercise options including flat, incline, and decline styles.

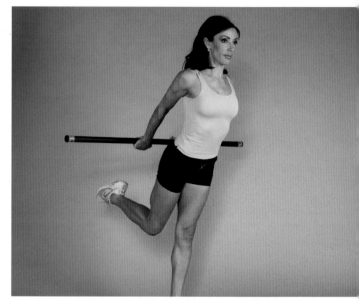

Bio-electrical impedance analysis scale A method for body composition analysis.

Biomechanically (sound) Referring to the mechanics of the human body. In this case, being of good structure and function.

Body Bar A solid-steel fitness bar encased in rubber. Body Bars come in predetermined weights with color-coded identification labels.

Body composition The proportion of fat to lean muscle mass in your body.

Body mass index (BMI) A measure of the relative amount of fat and muscle in the human body. BMI is calculated by dividing your weight in kilograms (kg) by your height in meters (m) squared. This can be expressed as BMI = kg / (m x m), where 1 kg = 2.2 lb and 1 m = 39.4 in. The healthy BMI range is 20 to 25. Above 25 is overweight, and above 30 is obese.

Body-weight exercises Exercises that use all or part of your body weight for resistance. Push-ups and sit-ups are examples of body-weight exercises.

BOSU Short for "Both Sides Up," the BOSU Balance Trainer is an inflated thick-rubber dome on a flat, 25-inch round platform.

Cable crossover machine A total body-weight training machine that uses cables to allow a full range of motion. Cable crossover machines typically use weight stacks to provide resistance.

Cable-motion system An exercise system that uses cables to allow an increased range of motion. Cable-motion systems typically use weight stacks to provide resistance.

Calorie A calorie is the metric unit of heat measurement. When used in relation to nutrition, it refers to the energy value of food, or the amount of energy used when performing an exercise.

Carbohydrates (carbs) Commonly and somewhat erroneously called sugars or starches. Carbohydrate-rich foods include bread, cookies, rice, potatoes, grains, and beans.

Cardiovascular system The body's system that moves nutrients, gases, and wastes to and from cells using blood in the veins and arteries of the circulatory system. This system also helps fight diseases and stabilizes body temperature.

Cardiovascular training (cardio) Also called *aerobic exercise* or *cardiovascular conditioning*, cardio conditions the heart and respiratory system. It increases your capacity to work, burns fat, and helps keep fat off your body.

Cellulite A condition in which the skin of the lower limbs, abdomen, and pelvic region becomes dimpled. This is caused by underlying fat cells bulging toward the skin layers.

Certified personal trainer A qualified professional fitness trainer, most commonly accredited by the American Council on Exercise (ACE).

Cholesterol A fat-based substance essential for cell health. Cholesterol is produced in the body and absorbed from foods. Too much cholesterol can build up on the artery walls, causing stroke and other circulatory problems.

Complex carbohydrates (complex carbs) Large-molecule, complicated carbohydrates that are digested more slowly than simple carbs and provide a slow, steady stream of energy. These are found in fruits, vegetables, nuts, seeds, grains, bread, cereal, rice, pasta, potatoes, and beans.

Compound movement Exercises that work two or more muscle groups simultaneously.

Compound stretching Engaging multiple muscles when stretching, especially large muscle groups.

Compression of morbidity The practice of living disease free and illness free for as long as possible.

Concentric contraction A muscular contraction where the muscle shortens (contracts) as you move it.

Cooldown The final phase of a workout. Cooldowns are used to slow your heart rate and help transition your body to its regular rhythm.

Core Also called *core muscles,* the core includes the major muscles of the abdomen, mid back, and low back.

Cortisol A hormone that increases blood pressure and blood sugar and reduces immune responses. Often referred to as a stress hormone, cortisol inhibits the body's ability to recover and can lead to overtraining.

Cross-training A combination of two or more types of physical activity. Cross-training helps keep you interested in exercise, giving your mind, muscles, and joints a break from repetitive stresses. It also facilitates recovery of the muscle groups not being worked.

Delayed-onset muscle soreness (DOMS) Also called *muscle fever,* DOMS is discomfort felt twenty-four to seventy-two hours after exercising. It is associated with muscle cell damage and micro-tears in the muscle fibers.

Delt The deltoid muscle.

Dumbbell A weight that can be held in one hand.

Eccentric contraction A muscular contraction where the muscle lengthens (extends) as you move it.

Elastic toners (toners) Tubes of elastic used to build strength and muscle tone. Oxygenfit toners are designed with a patented Soft-Touch Safety sleeve and comfortable handles for working out.

Electro muscle stimulation (e-stim) An electrical device that uses an electrical current (stimulation) to make muscle fibers contract. E-stim, also known as EMS, is used in the medical rehabilitation of wasted muscles and for physical training.

Elliptical trainer A type of low-impact training machine used for cardiovascular exercise.

Endorphin Naturally occurring neurotransmitters found in the brain and nervous system. Endorphins have opiate-like properties, relieving pain and creating a feeling of well-being.

Endurance training Exercising to increase stamina and endurance.

Equilibrioception Your sense of balance.

Extension To straighten out, or move to a position of full length.

Extensor Muscle used to extend; for example, the triceps on the upper arm.

External rotation Rotary motion away from the midline.

Fad diet Popular but scientifically unsound or unproven, fad diets promise quick results and are relatively easy to implement. They rarely promote sound weight loss and only work short-term, if at all.

Fixators Muscles that stabilize the bone in order to perform a movement. Fixators prevent unnecessary motion of other muscles and stabilizers. They help maintain alignment through movement and provide balance.

Flexibility The capacity for a joint to move freely through a full range of motion.

Flexion The bending of a limb or joint by the action of a flexor muscle.

Flexor Muscle that cause flexion; for example, the biceps on the upper arm.

Food and Drug Administration (FDA) An agency of the Department of Health and Human Services of the U.S. government. It regulates the use of food, drugs, medical devices, and related products.

FreeMotion Fitness machines An adjustable-cable machine that uses two cables to provide upper-body resistance through a full range of motion.

Free weight A weight, such as a barbell or dumbbell, that is not constrained or attached to another device.

Frontal plane Also called the *coronal plane,* this divides the body into front and back halves.

Functional fitness Training designed to improve the movements used in everyday life.

Functional fitness equipment Equipment used specifically for functional fitness training; may include Wobble boards, medicine balls, yoga blocks, elastic toners, Kettlebells, stability discs (or pillows), and Gliding discs.

Glider A sliding disc used in an exercise system that transforms movements into smooth, graceful lines of flowing motion.

Glutes Gluteus maximus muscle.

Gram (g) Unit of mass equal to 1/1000th of a kilogram. 1 ounce = 28 grams and 1 pound = 454 grams.

Heart rate monitor (HRM) An electrical device that measures your heart rate by sensing the electrical impulses produced by your heart. Heart rate monitors are usually incorporated in a wristwatch and use a chest strap to sense the impulses.

HDL High-density lipoproteins (HDLs) enable your body to move fats and cholesterol within the bloodstream. They are also thought to remove damaging plaque from the artery walls, aiding in the prevention of heart disease.

Hold move An exercise move where you hold a position for a predetermined length of time.

Holistic movement Taking into account the whole body as a system, not just its isolated parts.

Holistic stretching A mixture of yoga and Chinese healing used to increase health and wellness.

Horizontal plane Also called the *transverse plane,* this divides the body horizontally into upper and lower halves.

Hormone A naturally occurring chemical messenger that transports signals from one cell to another.

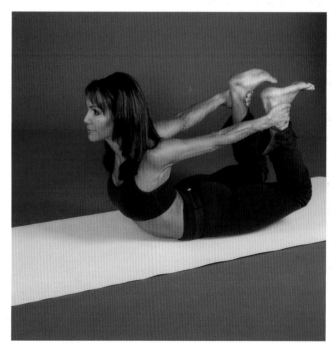

Hyperextension The position of a joint or a part of the body extending beyond the normal range of motion.

Internal rotation Rotary motion toward the midline.

Isometric exercise A type of strength training in which you don't change the position of the exercising muscles during contraction. The exercise is done in static a position so that the muscles either work against an immovable object or are held in a static position against other muscles.

Kilogram (kg) International unit of mass. 1 kilogram = 35 ounces or 2.2 pounds.

Kinesiology Also known as *human kinetics*, this is the study of human movement and biomechanics.

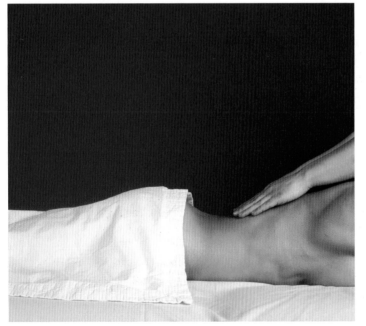

Lateral Toward the outside or side of the body.

Lats Latissimus dorsi muscle.

LDL Low-density lipoproteins (LDLs) enable your body to move fat and cholesterol within the bloodstream. High levels of LDLs are an indicator of medical problems like heart disease.

Lean body mass The amount of muscle in your body, especially skeletal muscle.

Massage The practice of soft-tissue manipulation using pressure, tension, motion, or vibration. Massage is used to work on muscles, tendons, ligaments, skin, joints, lymphatic vessels, and the gastrointestinal system. It can be applied with the hands, fingers, elbows, forearms, and feet.

Maximum heart rate (MHR) Your maximum heart rate is the highest rate at which your heart can possibly beat. It can be estimated by subtracting your age in years from 220.

Medial Toward the midline or middle of the body.

Median plane Also called the *sagital plane,* divides the body down the middle into left and right halves.

Metabolism, metabolic processes Metabolism is the group of chemical reactions that occur in your body to maintain life. These metabolic processes allow you to grow and reproduce, maintain tissues and organs, and function effectively.

Meter (m) International unit of length. 1 meter = 39.4 inches.

Muscle definition The visible outline of muscle through the skin.

Musculoskeletal system Also known as the *locomotor system,* this is the system of muscles and bones that together allow us to move.

Naturally Caffeinated A state of high energy, enthusiasm, and enjoyment of life.

Neutral stance Also known as the *anatomical position,* this is used as a reference when describing parts of the body in relation to each other. Neutral stance is standing erect with the head, eyes, and toes pointing forward and feet together with arms by the sides. The palms of the hands also point forward.

Obliques The external oblique and internal oblique muscles.

Olympic bar A metal bar that is 7.22 feet long and weights 44.1 pounds. The Olympic bar is the standard used in competitive weightlifting.

Osteoporosis Bone condition characterized by a decrease in density and an increase in porosity and brittleness.

Overtraining Training too much or too often or when you fail to get enough recovery in between workouts.

Pecs Pectoralis major muscles. The fan-shaped muscles located on the upper front of the chest wall.

Pedometer A small electronic device used to measure speed, distance, number of steps, and calories burned while walking or running. Pedometers are often incorporated with wristwatches.

Pilates A no-impact exercise routine that stretches and lengthens the major muscle groups without neglecting the smaller muscles. Pilates emphasizes body alignment and correct breathing.

Planes of motion A system for describing the body's movement in three perpendicular planes—the frontal, lateral, and medial. The planes of motion describe movement relative to your body at a neutral stance.

Plate-loaded machine A weight-training machine that uses plates loaded on a barbell.

Plié (pronounced *plee-ay*) A movement where you lower your body, bending the knees outward in line with the out-turned feet.

Plyometrics A type of exercise training designed to produce fast, powerful movements and improve the functions of the nervous system. Plyometrics may include jumping, bounding, and hopping exercises.

Posterior To the back; for example, the posterior deltoid is on the back of your shoulder.

Prime movers The large muscles in your body that provide the bulk of the power when you perform a movement.

Prone Lying down, on your back.

Proprioception The ability to sense the position, location, orientation, and movement of the body.

Proprioceptive neuromuscular facilitation (PNF) A method of stretching that alternates between an assisted passive stretch and an isometric stretch of the same muscle.

Proprioceptor A sensory receptor, found primarily in muscles, tendons, joints, and the inner ear, that detects the motion and position of the body.

Protein A complex organic compound essential for the chemical processes that sustain life. Dietary protein is found in foods such as meat, fish, and eggs.

Range of motion The distance between the fully flexed position and fully extended position of a joint or muscle group.

Reps The number of repetitions of an exercise movement in a "set." One rep is a complete exercise cycle; for example, one biceps curl.

Resistance bands Large elastic bands, often with handles, used as a total-body training system.

Resistance exercise See *resistance training.*

Resistance training A form of training in which muscular effort is performed against an opposing force. The goal of resistance training is to gradually and progressively overload the musculoskeletal system so it gets stronger.

Respiratory system The body system for breathing. It includes the lungs and airways.

Ripped The state of having highly defined muscles and low body fat, also described as *cut.*

Runner's high A feeling of exhilaration resulting from intense exercise, often called an *endorphin rush.*

Selectorized machines Weight-training machines that allow you to select the amount of weight being used.

Set A group of repeated exercises, or reps; for example, a set of twelve biceps curls.

Six pack Highly defined abdominal muscles.

Skeletal muscle The muscles that attach to bones, usually via tendons. Skeletal muscle is contracted voluntarily (by thinking about it) unlike cardiac (heart) muscle and the smooth muscle of the digestive tract that act without conscious thought.

Smith machine An apparatus that constrains a barbell to move only upward and downward. Some Smith machines allow limited forward and backward movement.

Spot reducing A mythical belief that it is possible to loose fat in an isolated area by exercising that particular area.

Squat cage Also known as a *power cage, power rack,* or *squat rack,* the squat cage increases safety when using a barbell.

Stability ball An exercise ball, also known as a *Swiss ball,* made of soft, durable plastic with a diameter of 35 to 85 centimeters (14 to 34 inches).

Stabilizer muscles The smaller peripheral muscles that provide stabilization and support for your joints and movements.

Stationary bike A machine that simulates the motion of cycling. Stationary bikes can be a real bicycle attached to a stand that lifts the back wheel off the ground.

Strength training The use of resistance to build the strength, muscular endurance, and tone of skeletal muscles. There are many different methods of strength training. The most common is the use of metal weights or elastic/hydraulic forces to provide resistance.

Subcutaneous fat Body fat that lies just beneath the skin. Subcutaneous fat can be measured using body fat calipers to give an approximation of total body fat.

Superset A training technique combining two or more consecutive exercises with little or no rest in between.

Supersetalicious A highly pleasing superset, affording great enjoyment once completed.

Supination Rolling or rotating to the outside.

Supine Lying facedown, on your front.

T-bar A seated exercise machine used to exercise your back muscles.

Target heart rate range The minimum and maximum heart rate in beats per minute (BPM) between which you want to train. Target heart rate range varies depending on your training goals.

Testosterone A naturally occurring steroid hormone that aids in growth, muscular development, health, well-being, and sexual function. Testosterone enhances libido and energy levels, aids in the production of red blood cells, and protects against osteoporosis.

Traps Trapezius muscle.

TVA Transversus abdominis. The group of muscles that run laterally from your sides to the front of your body.

Unconscious competence The ability to perform tasks without having to think about them.

Unilateral One side only.

Vinyasa A flowing, dynamic form of yoga that focuses on the journey between multiple postures, not just the individual postures.

VMO Vastus medialis oblique muscle.

Warm-up Light exercise used to increase body temperature, blood flow, respiration, and metabolic processes in preparation for more intense training.

Weight-bearing exercise Exercise that requires you to support or lift your own body weight. Examples include running, walking, dancing, elliptical training machines, stair climbing, yoga, and Pilates.

Weight plate A weighted disc, usually made of metal, which is placed on a barbell. Multiple plates are used on a bar to increase weight.

Weight-stack machine An exercise machine that uses a stack of weights for resistance. Typical weight-stack machines employ a system of cables, levers, or other mechanisms to transfer the load to the user.

Wobble board An unstable platform that you stand on to promote balance, coordination, body awareness, core strength, and stability. Other varieties of stability board include the balance board and rocker board.

Yoga A system of exercises practiced as part of a Hindu philosophy to promote control of the body and mind.

INDEX

INDEX